Student Workbook

to Accompany

D1560696

Calculating Drug Dosages: An Interactive Approach to Learning Nursing Math

SECOND EDITION

Sandra Luz Martinez de Castillo, RN, MA, EdD

Nursing Instructor
Contra Costa College
San Pablo, California

and

Maryanne Werner-McCullough, RN, MS, MNP

Nursing Instructor
Contra Costa College
San Pablo, California

F. A. Davis Company • Philadelphia

F. A. Davis Company
1915 Arch Street
Philadelphia, PA 19103
www.fadavis.com

ISBN-10:   0-8036-1673-2
ISBN-13:   978-0-8036-1673-8

Printed in the United States of America

Last digit indicates print number: 10 9 8 7 6 5

Publisher, Nursing: Robert G. Martone
Associate Acquisitions Editor: Tom Ciavarella
Design Manager: Carolyn O'Brien

NOTE: Author and publisher have done everything possible to ensure content herein is accurate, current, and in accord with accepted standards at the time of publication, and to secure permission to reproduce drug labels. The reader is advised that information related to drugs, including facsimiles of drug labels, is presented for demonstration purposes only, to illustrate calculation methods. The reader is further advised to refer to current pharmaceutical references for information about drug therapy and always check product information (package inserts) for new information regarding dose and contraindications before administering any drug. Caution is especially urged when using new or infrequently ordered drugs.

A Note to the Student

Dear Student:

Knowing how to calculate drug dosages accurately is a critical component of nursing practice. At first glance, learning all of the nursing math concepts may seem overwhelming. However, learning the math concepts presented in the CD-ROM and Student Workbook will help you develop strong nursing math skills. Further, applying the math concepts to common clinical situations will help you solve drug dosage problems competently and with confidence. The CD-ROM and Student Workbook are designed to make learning nursing math fun and easy.

In the second edition of *Calculating Drug Dosages: An Interactive Approach to Learning Nursing Math* CD-ROM, you will find 13 modules. Each module is developed to address the most common math concepts used in nursing practice. Within each module you will find:

- A tutorial of each math concept
- Critical thinking word problems
- Interactive learning activities
- Practice problems to help you apply the math concepts
- A choice of method (linear ratio and proportion, fractional ratio and proportion, dimensional analysis, and formula method) for solving problems
- Feedback on how to solve problems
- Section quizzes at the end of each math concept
- A module review covering all the math concepts presented in the module, with answers
- Two module tests that allow you to print out your score after completion of the test

NEW! ◆ Focus on Safety sections to highlight clinical situations and help avoid common errors

NEW! ◆ A new Preparation for NCLEX module that provides practice problems based on the format of the NCLEX licensure examination

NEW! ◆ Sections on High Alert Medications that link to information from Davis' Drug Guide

NEW! ◆ Updated medication labels, approved abbreviations, and units of measurement

The Student Workbook is designed to give you extra practice with the math concepts presented in the CD-ROM. More math problems are included in the Student Workbook, along with Focus on Safety exercises that require you to make clinical judgments/decisions. Answers are provided in the back of the book.

We hope that you will enjoy learning the nursing math concepts as you develop competency in solving drug dosage problems.

Sandra and Maryanne

Contents

FRACTIONS

KEY POINTS:
- Check the denominators before adding and subtracting fractions. If they are different, find the lowest common denominator, then solve the problem.
- For multiplication of fractions, just multiply the numerators and the denominators.
- For division of fractions, remember to invert the second fraction. Then, multiply the numerators and the denominators.
- Change all mixed numbers to improper fractions before working out the problem.
- Reduce all fractions to their lowest terms.

Working With Addition of Fractions
Add the following fractions and mixed numbers.

1. 2/5 + 1/5 = _____

2. 2/21 + 18/42 = _____

3. 2/5 + 2/3 = _____

4. 4 4/8 + 3/4 = _____

5. 2 3/4 + 1/5 + 2 1/2 = _____

6. 3 1/8 + 4 5/6 + 7 1/4 = _____

7. 8 2/9 + 2 1/5 + 3 2/3 = _____

8. $6\ 7/15 + 3\ 4/5 + 4\ 5/6$ = _____

9. $3\ 1/10 + 5\ 2/5 + 9\ 1/8$ = _____

10. $11\ 1/8 + 7\ 3/4 + 2\ 7/8$ = _____

Working With Subtraction of Fractions
Subtract the following fractions and mixed numbers.

1. $5/6 \quad - \quad 1/3$ = _____

2. $8/10 \quad - \quad 1/2$ = _____

3. $7/8 \quad - \quad 2/3$ = _____

4. $4\ 1/4 \quad - \quad 1\ 3/8$ = _____

5. $10\ 1/2 \quad - \quad 3\ 1/5$ = _____

6. $8\ 1/6 \quad - \quad 5\ 2/3$ = _____

7. $11\ 2/5 \quad - \quad 6\ 7/8$ = _____

8. $20\ 1/8 \quad - \quad 9\ 2/3$ = _____

9. $15\ 2/7 \quad - \quad 4\ 5/6$ = _____

10. $10\ 1/2 \quad - \quad 3\ 2/5$ = _____

Working With Multiplication of Fractions
Multiply the following fractions and mixed numbers.

1. 6/8 x 2/5 = _____

2. 10/9 x 1/2 = _____

3. 5/12 x 1 1/5 = _____

4. 3 1/8 x 3/10 = _____

5. 5 1/2 x 3 3/5 = _____

6. 3 1/3 x 4 3/7 = _____

7. 2 5/6 x 1 1/8 = _____

8. 4 5/7 x 2 2/5 = _____

9. 6 1/8 x 3 2/3 = _____

10. 1 1/9 x 2 11/12 = _____

Working With Division of Fractions
Divide the following fractions and mixed numbers.

1. 7/10 ÷ 1/2 = _____

2. 1/150 ÷ 1/3 = _____

3. 6/8 ÷ 3/5 = _____

4. 4 5/7 ÷ 1/2 = _____

5. 3 1/2 ÷ 3 3/4 = _____

6. 2 2/5 ÷ 5 4/5   = _____

7. 4 1/8 ÷ 7 1/2   = _____

8. 6 2/9 ÷ 3 1/3   = _____

9. 4 5/7 ÷ 1/7   = _____

10. 5 1/2 ÷ 8 3/4   = _____

DECIMALS

KEY POINTS:
- **When adding and subtracting decimals, make sure that the decimal points are lined up correctly.**
- **For multiplication of decimals, count the total number of decimal places in the numbers to be multiplied. Then, count the same number of decimal places in the answer and place the decimal point.**
- **When dividing decimals, if there is a decimal point in the divisor, move the decimal point to make the divisor a whole number. Then, move the decimal point in the dividend the same number of decimal places. Place the decimal point in the answer in the same place as in the dividend.**

Working With Addition of Decimals
Add the following decimals.

1. $3.7 + 5998 + 0.0032 + 72.91 =$ _____

2. $78.2 + 55 + 9.005$ = _____

3. $1.75 + 0.234 + 0.004$ = _____

4. $0.17 + 7 + 1954 + 0.0013$ = _____

5.   2.29 + 5.01 + 45 + 4.67 = _____

6.   53.1 + 8.2 + 9.5 = _____

7.   11.6 + 10 + 0.02 = _____

8.   2.17 + 7.1 + 50 + 0.25 = _____

9.   20.4 + 0.1 + 37 + 8.21 = _____

10.   3.09 + 6.70 + 5 + 14.2 = _____

11.   31.4 + 2.1 + 1.09 + 1.4 = _____

12.   0.07 + 4.25 + 19 + 4.8 = _____

Working With Subtraction of Decimals
Subtract the following decimals.

1.   321.02 − 0.0045 = _____

2.   1.031 − 0.98 = _____

3.   9012.4 − 0.067 = _____

4.   7050.3 − 1.037 = _____

5.   8 − 0.023 = _____

6.   605.1 − 4.05 = _____

7.   425.2 − 1.503 = _____

8.   67.09 − 0.29 = _____

9.   9167.3 − 463.5 = _____

10.   876 − 22.9 = _____

11.   1256.3 − 702.4 = _____

12.   950 − 10.8   = _____

Working With Multiplication of Decimals
Multiply the following decimals.

1.   301.12 x   0.25   = _____

2.   2.021   x   0.8   = _____

3.   502.6   x   0.67   = _____

4.   75.3   x   1.037   = _____

5.   5.1   x   0.02   = _____

6.   201.01 x   0.15   = _____

7.   61.48   x   0.06   = _____

8.   30.6   x   0.24   = _____

9.   150   x   2.134   = _____

10. 8.25   x   0.03   = _____

11. 65.02   x   1.04   = _____

12. 10.3   x   4.9   = _____

Working With Division of Decimals
Divide the following decimals.

1.   0.9   ÷   0.02   = _____

2.   16.80   ÷   0.15   = _____

3.   382.32 ÷   54   = _____

4.   75.85   ÷   3.7   = _____

5.   0.0015 ÷ 0.03   = _____

6.   100.3 ÷ 0.25   = _____

7.   250.12 ÷ 5.2   = _____

8.   1000.8 ÷ 12   = _____

9.   70.05 ÷ 1.5   = _____

10.   0.0226 ÷ 0.4   = _____

11.   618.2 ÷ 12.5   = _____

12.   0.542 ÷ 0.5   = _____

ROMAN NUMERALS

KEY POINTS:
- Read roman numerals from left to right.
- Remember the following rules:
    - The roman numerals I, X, C, and M may be repeated in sequence, but only up to three times.
    - The roman numerals V, L, and D may never be repeated in sequence.
    - A smaller numeral to the right of a larger numeral is added to the larger numeral.
    - A smaller numeral to the left of a larger numeral is subtracted from the larger numeral.

Working With Roman Numerals
Write the roman numerals for the following arabic numbers.

1. 7 1/2   = _____

2. 35   = _____

3. 41   = _____

4. 65   = _____

5. 101   = _____

6. 15 1/2   = _____

7. 99   = _____

8. 2011   = _____

Write the arabic numbers for the following roman numerals.

1. XXX = _____

2. XIV = _____

3. XLIX = _____

4. ISS = _____

5. CL = _____

6. XCV = _____

7. LXXV = _____

8. MMX = _____

Module: METHODS OF CALCULATION

SELECT A METHOD OF CALCULATION

Linear Ratio and Proportion:
$$5 \text{ mg} : 1 \text{ tab} :: 10 \text{ mg} : x \text{ tab}$$

Fractional Ratio and Proportion:
$$\frac{5 \text{ mg}}{1 \text{ tab}} = \frac{10 \text{ mg}}{x \text{ tab}}$$

Dimensional Analysis:
$$\frac{10 \text{ mg}}{1} \times \frac{1 \text{ tab}}{5 \text{ mg}} = x \text{ tab}$$

Formula:
$$\frac{10 \text{ mg}}{5 \text{ mg}} \times 1 \text{ tab} = x \text{ tab}$$

KEY POINTS:
- Learn the method of your choice; study the setup.
- To arrive at the correct answer, the units of measurement must be set up so that they cancel.

Working With a Method of Calculation
Solve the following problems using the method of your choice.

1. The order is for 50 mg. The pharmacy sends 25 mg tablets. How many tablets will the nurse give?

   _____

2. The order is for 75 mg. The pharmacy sends 50 mg scored tablets. How many tablets will the nurse give?

   _____

3. The order is for 1 mcg. The pharmacy sends 0.5 mcg pills. How many pills will the nurse give?

_____

4. The order is for 0.5 g. The pharmacy sends 1 g scored tablets. How many tablets will the nurse give?

_____

5. The order is for 1.2 gram. The pharmacy sends 0.4 gram caplets. How many caplets will the nurse give?

_____

6. The order is for 7 mg. The pharmacy sends an elixir labeled 2 mg / mL. How many mL will the nurse give?

_____

7. The order is for 90 mg of a drug. The pharmacy sends 30 mg / 2 mL. How many mL will the nurse give?

_____

8. The doctor orders Lanoxin 125 mcg daily. The nurse finds the following in the patient's medication drawer. How many mL of Lanoxin will the nurse administer?

Lanoxin
500 mcg per 2 mL

_____

9. The order is for IV ranitidine 75 mg q.8h. The pharmacy sends the following vial of ranitidine. How many mL will the nurse give?

```
Ranitidine for Injection

25 mg / mL
```

_____

10. The order is for 100 mg. The pharmacy sends an oral suspension labeled 12.5 mg / 2 mL. How many mL will the nurse give?

_____

11. The order is for amoxicillin/clavulanate 250 mg t.i.d. The pharmacy sends the following medication. How many days will the bottle last?

```
Amoxicillin/Clavulanate
Potassium Tablets

250 mg / tablet

Contains 30 tablets
```

_____

12. The order is for 125 mg b.i.d. The pharmacy sends a 200 mL bottle labeled 12.5 mg / mL. How many days will the bottle last?

_____

13. The order is for 0.015 gram of medication IM stat. The pharmacy sends a vial of the medication labeled 0.01 gram per 1.5 mL. How many mL will the nurse administer?

_____

14. The physician orders 21 mg p.o. t.i.d. The nurse has a 100 mL bottle labeled 6 mg / mL. How much will the patient receive?

_____

15. The patient is to receive 60 mcg p.o. q.AM. The nurse has a bottle labeled 4 mcg / 2 mL. How many mL will the patient receive each day?

_____

16. The physician orders heparin sodium 6000 units subcut q.12h. The pharmacy sends the following vial of heparin. How many mL will the patient receive per dose?

```
Heparin Sodium
10,000 units / mL
```

_____

17. The doctor orders 0.4 mg of a drug b.i.d. The pharmacy sends a bottle labeled 0.4 mg per pill. The bottle contains 30 pills. How many days will this bottle last?

_____

18. The patient has an order for amoxicillin oral suspension 500 mg q.8h. The medication drawer contains the following bottle of amoxicillin. How many mL will the patient receive per dose?

```
+-----------------------------------------------+
|                                               |
|   Amoxicillin Oral Suspension                 |
|                                               |
|      +-----------------------------+          |
|      |     125 mg in 5 mL          |          |
|      +-----------------------------+          |
|                                               |
|   For oral use only. Shake well before use.   |
|                                               |
+-----------------------------------------------+
```

_____

19a. The doctor orders 0.4 mg of a medication b.i.d. The pharmacy sends a vial labeled 1 mg / mL. How many mL will the patient receive?

_____

b. If the vial contains 2 mL, how many doses are available in the vial?

_____

20a. The order is for heparin 8000 units subcut now. The pharmacy sends the following dose of heparin. Calculate the number of mL the patient will receive.

> # Heparin Sodium
>
> ## 10,000 units / mL
>
> Multidose vial containing 4 mL

_____

b. How many doses will the nurse be able to give from the above vial?

_____

c. If the order is changed to heparin 6500 units subcut daily, how many mL will the patient receive per dose?

_____

d. How many doses of the above order would the nurse be able to give from the vial?

_____

Module: SYSTEMS OF MEASUREMENT

METRIC SYSTEM:
UNITS OF MEASUREMENT

Kilo Hecto Deka BASIC Deci Centi Milli Micro
UNIT

KEY POINTS:
- Memorize the metric units of measurement, metric abbreviations, and the metric line.

Working With the Metric System
Fill in the blanks with the correct answer.

1.	3.500 L	= _____	mL
2.	0.7 L	= _____	mL
3.	1000 mg	= _____	gram
4.	100 mcg	= _____	mg
5.	10 mg	= _____	mcg
6.	2 mg	= _____	mcg
7.	35.6 mg	= _____	gram
8.	7.45 mL	= _____	L
9.	0.07 cm	= _____	dm
10.	10 km	= _____	m
11.	100 cm	= _____	mm
12.	1.65 kg	= _____	g

13. 1500 mL = _____ L

14. 2.5 g = _____ mg

15. The patient receives vancomycin 750 mg IV b.i.d. How many g does the patient receive per dose?

    _____

16. The patient has an order for 0.5 g of ampicillin. How many mg will the nurse administer?

    _____

17. The patient receives levothyroxine 75 mcg p.o. q.AM. How many mg does the patient receive?

    _____

18. The doctor's order is for digoxin elixir 0.45 mg p.o. now. This dose is equivalent to ____ mcg.

    _____

19. The weight of a medication is 1.2 kg. This is equivalent to __ g.

    _____

20. A wound measures 4 cm in length. This is equivalent to ____ mm.

    _____

21. The patient has an order for Versed® 7 mg IV for the patient. The pharmacy sends a vial of Versed labeled 5 mg / mL. How many mL will the nurse administer?

    _____

22. The drug order is for lactulose 1000 mg p.o. b.i.d. for the patient. The pharmacy sends a container labeled lactulose 1 g / 10 mL. How many mL will the nurse administer per dose?

_____

23. The doctor orders Solu-Medrol® 125 mg IV q.12h for the patient. The pharmacy sends Solu-Medrol 0.25 g / mL. How many mL will the nurse administer per dose?

_____

24. The physician writes an order for Benadryl® 50 mg orally q.6h. as needed for the patient. The nurse has a bottle of Benadryl labeled 12.5 mg / 5 mL. How many mL will the nurse administer per dose?

_____

25. The nurse is preparing to administer 750 mg of Vitamin C to the patient at 9:00 AM. In the patient's medication drawer, the nurse finds Vitamin C tablets labeled 0.5 g / tablet. How many tablets will the nurse administer to the patient at 9:00 AM?

_____

26. The patient has an order for lorazepam 0.5 mg IM now. The nurse has lorazepam labeled 2 mg / mL. How many mL will the nurse administer to the patient?

_____

HOUSEHOLD SYSTEM:
UNITS OF MEASUREMENT

UNIT	EQUIVALENT MEASUREMENT	ABBREVIATION
1 glass	8 ounces	--
1 cup	8 ounces	--
1 teacup	6 ounces	--
1 tablespoon	3 teaspoons	T, Tbs
1 teaspoon	5 mL	t, tsp
1 drop (drops)	1 minim	gt (gtt)
2.2 pounds	1 kilogram	lb

KEY POINTS:

- Memorize the units of measurement, equivalent measurements, and symbols used in the household system.

Working With the Household System
Fill in the blanks with the correct answer.

1. Two Tbs = _____ tsp

2. One ounce = _____ T

3. One-half ounce = _____ tsp

4. Two glasses of juice = _____ oz

5. One cup = _____ oz

6. 2 kg = _____ lb

7. Three tsp of an antacid = _____ T.
   Fill in the medicine cup below.

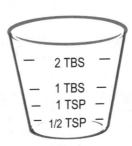

8. The nurse administers 2 tsp of cough syrup to the patient. How many mL will the nurse administer?

   _____

   Fill in the medicine cup below.

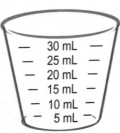

9. The patient drinks 3 glasses of water. How many ounces did the patient drink?

   _____

10. The nurse gives the patient a cup of broth. How many ounces is this?

   _____

CONVERSIONS BETWEEN SYSTEMS:
UNITS OF MEASUREMENT

UNIT		EQUIVALENT MEASUREMENTS	
1 inch	=	2.54 cm	
1 oz	=	30 mL	= 2 T
1 tsp	=	5 mL	
1 T	=	15 mL	= 3 tsp
1 glass	=	8 ounces	= 240 mL
1 cup	=	8 ounces	= 240 mL
1 teacup	=	6 ounces	= 180 mL
1 gt	=	1 minim	
16 minims	=	1 mL	
2.2 lb	=	1 kilogram	

KEY POINTS:
- Memorize the equivalent measurements for the metric and household systems of measurement.

Working With Conversions Between Systems
Fill in the blanks with the correct answer.

1. 1/2 oz = ____mL

2. 1 mcg = ____mg

3. 2 T = ____oz

4. 0.03 mg = ____mcg

5. 1.75 g = ____mg

6. 0.5 g = ____mg

7. 45 mL = ____oz

8. 25 mL = ____tsp

9. 85 mg = ____g

10. 32 min = ____mL

11. 20 mL = ____t

12. 3 T = ____t

13. 2 cups = ____mL

14. 1 inch = ____cm

15. 1 cm = ____mm

16. 75 kg = ____lb

17. 198 lb = ____kg

18. 3 dL = ____L

19. The doctor orders thyroxine 0.2 mg p.o. for the patient. Thyroxine is available in 100 mg tablets. How many tablets will the nurse give?

_____

20. The patient drinks two 6 oz cups of coffee for breakfast. How many mL did the patient drink?

_____

21. A patient weighs 84 kg. How many pounds does the patient weigh?

_____

22. Order: cephalexin 500 mg
    Available: cephalexin 0.25 gram per tablet

    How many tablets will the nurse give?

_____

23. The physician orders Roxanol® 30 mg p.o. q.3h. p.r.n. for pain for the patient. Roxanol is available in a bottle labeled 10 mg / 5 mL. How many tsp will the nurse administer?

_____

24. The patient has an order to administer 600 mcg of a drug subcut to the patient. The pharmacy sends an ampule labeled 2 mg / mL. How many mL will the nurse administer?

_____

25. The nurse has an order to administer 75 mg of meperidine hydrochloride IM now. In the narcotic drawer, the nurse finds an ampule of meperidine hydrochloride labeled 100 mg / mL. How many mL will the nurse administer?

_____

Module: INTAKE AND OUTPUT

INTAKE AND OUTPUT:
EQUIVALENT MEASUREMENTS

1 glass	8 ounces	240 mL
1 cup	8 ounces	240 mL
1 teacup	6 ounces	180 mL
1 styrofoam cup	6 ounces	180 mL
1 popsicle	3 ounces	90 mL

ice cubes   (melt to ½ the original volume)

1 ounce (oz)	30 mL
1 tablespoon (T, Tbs)	15 mL
1 teaspoon (t, tsp)	5 mL

KEY POINTS:
- Intake and output (I & O) are calculated in mL.
- The size of food containers varies, so it is important for the nurse to become familiar with the specific containers used in each clinical setting.
- Parenteral intake is calculated as a part of the total intake.

Working With Intake and Output
Add the following intakes and outputs.

1.   The patient is on strict I & O. For breakfast, the patient took 1 cup of coffee, a 4 ounce glass of juice, and 240 mL of milk. For lunch, the patient had a styrofoam cup of tea and 6 ounces of broth. The patient voided 260 mL at 1000, and 180 mL at 1400. Calculate the patient's I & O.

I _____

O _____

2. The patient is n.p.o. for breakfast. For lunch, the patient was allowed to take 120 mL of water. The patient vomited 180 mL at 1300 and voided 100 mL at 1330. At 1400, the patient took 2 T of JELL-O® and ½ glass of apple juice. Calculate the patient's I & O.

I _____

O _____

3. The patient has a NG tube connected to low wall suction. At 0930, the MD wrote an order to clamp the NG tube. The nurse emptied 280 mL of NG drainage. At 1100, the patient vomited 325 mL of bile-colored drainage. The NG tube was reconnected to suction and drained an additional 475 mL by the end of the shift. The patient's wound drainage tube collected 60 mL of serosanguineous fluid. The patient's indwelling urinary catheter drained 270 mL of dark amber urine. Calculate the patient's output.

O _____

4. A patient who had prostate surgery yesterday has an indwelling urinary catheter with a continuous bladder irrigation. He is n.p.o. for breakfast and is started on a clear liquid diet for lunch. He took 6 ounces of broth and 4 ounces of cranberry juice. By the end of the shift, the nurse calculates that 2000 mL of bladder irrigant has infused. The total amount emptied from the urinary bag was 2270 mL. Calculate the I & O.

I _____

O _____

5.   The patient has an IV of D5W infusing at
       125 mL / hr. For breakfast, the patient took
       1 glass of juice and a cup of coffee. For lunch,
       the patient took six ounces of soup and a 12
       ounce can of soda. The patient voided 220 mL at
       1000 and 375 mL at 1400. Calculate the
       patient's 8-hr total I & O.

                        I _____
                        O _____

6.   At 0700, the patient is n.p.o. and has a primary
       IV of 1 L of D5NS q.10h, infusing continuously.
       The patient receives gentamicin 80 mg IVPB in
       100 mL NS at 0900 – 1700 – 0100, and
       metronidazole 500 mg in 100 mL NS at 0800.
       Calculate the patient's total parenteral intake
       starting at 0700 and ending at 1500.

                        I _____

7.   At 0700, the nurse started an IV of 1 L LR and
       set the infusion pump at 83 mL / hr. The patient
       was put on strict I & O. The patient was started
       on famotidine 20 mg IVPB in 50 mL NS, at 0800
       and 2000. For breakfast, the patient took 1 cup
       of coffee and a 6 ounce bowl of Cream of
       Wheat®. He was n.p.o. except for ice chips for
       the rest of the shift. The patient took 6 ounces of
       ice chips and voided 425 mL. Calculate the
       patient's total I & O starting at 0700 and ending
       at 1500.

                        I _____
                        O _____

8. At 1500, the patient had an IV of 1 L of D5W infusing at 125 mL / hr. For dinner, the patient took 1 glass of juice and an 8 ounce can of nutritional supplement. The IV infiltrated at 1800 and was restarted at 2000. The patient received KCl 20 mEq IVPB in 100 mL D5W at 1700. The patient voided twice for the entire shift (315 mL and 290 mL). Calculate the patient's total I & O starting at 1500 and ending at 2300.

I _____

O _____

9. At 2300, the patient had an IV of 1 L of 0.45% NS infusing at 50 mL / hr. The patient had coffee-ground emesis measuring 480 mL at 0100. The MD ordered 2 units of PRBCs over 3 hours, followed by an IV of 0.9% NS, to infuse at 150 mL / hr. The nurse discontinued the current IV and started the first unit of PRBC (250 mL) at 0200, and the second unit (270 mL) at 0330. The IV of 0.9% NS was started at 0500. Calculate the patient's total I & O starting at 2300 and ending at 0700.

I _____

O _____

10. At 1500, the patient had 900 mL left in the IV bag. The IV was infusing at 75 mL / hr. At 1900, the IV infiltrated and was restarted 1 hour later. The physician increased the IV rate to 125 mL / hr at 2000. Calculate the patient's total parenteral intake starting at 1500 and ending at 2300.

I _____

11.   At 0700, the MD ordered 1 L of D5/0.45% NS to infuse at 75 mL / hr for the first 3 hours, and then at 125 mL continuously. For breakfast, the patient took 1 cup of coffee, 8 ounces of milk and 6 ounces of orange juice. The patient voided 50 mL at 0900, and 75 mL at 1000. At 1100, the nurse inserted a Foley catheter per MD order and obtained 425 mL of urine. For lunch, the patient only took 5 ounces of broth. The nurse emptied the Foley catheter at 1500 and obtained 250 mL. Calculate the patient's total I & O starting at 0700 and ending at 1500.

I _____

O _____

12.   At 0900, the nurse begins the care of a patient who has just been transferred from the post-anesthesia care unit. The patient has a new liter of D5/0.9% NS infusing at 125 mL / hr. The patient has an indwelling urinary catheter with continuous bladder irrigation of NS infusing at 75 mL per hour, to keep the catheter free of clots. At 1500, the nurse empties 1575 mL from the urinary catheter. Calculate the patient's total I & O starting at 0900 and ending at 1500.

I _____

O _____

13.   At 2300, the patient had 850 mL left in the IV bag. The IV was infusing at 50 mL / hr. At 0200, the IV infiltrated and was restarted 2 hours later. The physician increased the IV rate to 75 mL / hr at 0400. Calculate the patient's total parenteral intake starting at 2300 and ending at 0700.

I _____

Exercise: FOCUS ON SAFETY
Making Clinical Judgments in Working With Intake and Output

- Read each situation, and then make a clinical judgment.
- Provide a rationale for your decision or action.

SITUATION:
The evening shift nurse learns during the change of shift report that the assigned patient is n.p.o., has a primary IV that has infused continuously all shift at 75 mL / hr, and received KCl 20 mEq in 100 mL NS at 0900 and 1300. In reviewing the patient's documented intake and output from the day shift, the evening nurse is most correct to:

Intake and Output

	Oral	IV	Urine	Emesis	Other
7 – 3	NPO	600 100	250 100 225		
Total mL	0	700	575		
3 – 11					

a. question the recorded 100 mL urine output.

c. question the documented amount of the IVPBs.

b. recalculate the primary IV intake.

d. plan to administer an IVPB of KCl.

Rationale / Discussion:

NASOGASTRIC TUBE FEEDING PROBLEMS

KEY POINTS:
- **Preparing dilute tube feedings requires calculating the number of mL of water to add to the formula to make the ordered strength.**
- **Information needed to solve the problem includes the amount of formula in the can and the ordered strength.**

Working With Nasogastric Tube Feeding Problems

1. The doctor orders a 3/4-strength formula tube feeding for the patient. The formula comes in cans containing 240 mL. How much water will the nurse add to the can of formula to make the ordered 3/4-strength diluted tube feeding?

   _____

2. The patient receives a 1/3-strength formula tube feeding. The formula can contains 233 mL. How much water will the nurse add to the can to make the 1/3-strength diluted tube feeding?

   _____

3. The order is to prepare a 2/3-strength tube feeding of Nepro® for a patient with a percutaneous endoscopic gastrostomy (PEG) tube. How much water will the nurse add to the 237 mL can of Nepro to make a 2/3-strength tube feeding?

   _____

4. The physician orders 200 mL of a 1/4-strength tube feeding q.6h., for a patient with a NG tube. The formula can contains 250 mL. How much water will the nurse add to make the 1/4-strength tube feeding?

   _____

5. A patient who has been receiving full-strength Jevity Plus® PEG tube feedings develops diarrhea. The physician orders a diluted tube feeding of 1/2-strength Jevity Plus for the patient. How much water will the nurse add to the 237 mL can of Jevity Plus to make a 1/2-strength tube feeding?

   _____

6. The physician orders a 1/4-strength tube feeding of Osmolite® at 40 mL / hr for a patient with a NG tube. The Osmolite can contains 237 mL. How much water will the nurse add to make a 1/4-strength tube feeding?

   _____

7. A patient has an order for 1/2-strength Pulmocare® tube feedings, at 50 mL / hr through a PEG tube. The nurse prepares the dilute formula and has a total volume of 475 mL. According to hospital policy, only 4 hours of tube feeding formula can be hung at a time, to minimize bacterial growth. How many mL of the prepared 1/2-strength formula will the nurse use?

   _____

8. The physician orders a 250 mL bolus N/G tube feeding of 3/4-strength tube feeding q.8h. The formula can contains 237 mL. How much water will the nurse add to make the 3/4-strength tube feeding?

   _____

9. The physician orders a diluted tube feeding of 1/3-strength Jevity Plus for the patient. How much water will the nurse add to the 250 mL can of Jevity Plus to make a 1/3-strength tube feeding?

   _____

10. The physician orders a 2/3-strength tube feeding of Suplena® at 25 mL / hr, for a patient with a nasogastric tube. The Suplena can contains 240 mL. How much water will the nurse add to make a 2/3-strength tube feeding?

    _____

Exercise: FOCUS ON SAFETY
Making Clinical Judgments in Working With Nasogastric Tube Feedings

- Read each situation, and then make a clinical judgment.
- Provide a rationale for your decision or action.

SITUATION:
The nurse adds 80 mL of water to 200 mL Jevity formula. The formula tube feeding is started to 0900 at the ordered rate. The patient has a primary IV of NS 0.9% infusing at 80 mL for the 8-hr shift. The nurse emptied 575 mL of urine at 1500, the end of the shift. Which nursing action requires follow up?

Date	Physician's Orders
2/12	Start N/G tube feeding of Jevity 2/3- strength at 50 mL per hour.
	Patient B ID *******

Intake and Output

	Oral	IV	Urine	Emesis	Foley
7 – 3	N/G				
Total mL	300	640			575
3 – 11					

a. The documented N/G tube intake should be 400 mL.

c. The IV intake is incorrect for the ordered rate.

b. The amount of water added to the formula.

d. The formula strength should be questioned.

Rationale / Discussion: _____

_____

_____

_____

_____

_____

Module: READING MEDICATION LABELS

READING MEDICATION LABELS

KEY POINTS:

- The essential information found on medication labels includes the following:
  - trade name
  - dosage strength
  - route of administration
  - instructions for mixing
  - generic name
  - form of the drug
  - expiration date
  - recommended dose

- The useful information found on medication labels includes the following:
  - total quantity
  - storage information
  - controlled substance symbol
  - manufacturer's name
  - lot number

Working With Reading Medication Labels
Use the medication labels to fill in the answers.

1.

Batch:
Expires:

K1A0

08637973   NDC 0026-2862-51

PRECOSE®
(acarbose tablets)

100 mg
100 Tablets

℞ Only

Bayer HealthCare
Bayer Pharmaceuticals Corporation
400 Morgan Lane
West Haven, CT 06516
Made in Germany

DESCRIPTION: Each tablet contains 100 mg acarbose.
DOSAGE: See accompanying literature for complete information on dosage and administration.
RECOMMENDED STORAGE: Do not store above 25°C (77°F). Protect from moisture. Keep container tightly closed.

N 3   0026-2862-51   5

06753701. R.2   12150   1003
©2003 Bayer Pharmaceuticals Corporation   Printed in USA

a. Trade name _____

b. Generic name _____

c. Dosage strength _____

d. Form of the drug _____

e. Routes of administration _____

2.

```
      0.5 mL        1 mL        1.5 mL        2 mL
  | | | | | | | | | | | | | | | | | | | | | | | | |

2 mL Carpuject®                NDC 0409-1276-32      RL-0742 (12/04)
Sterile Cartridge Unit with Luer Lock
Fentanyl Citrate Inj., USP  ℭⅡ   ‖‖‖‖‖‖‖‖‖‖‖‖‖‖‖‖‖‖
100 mcg Fentanyl / 2 mL
50 mcg per mL (0.05 mg per mL) ℞ only  (01) 0 030409 127632 1
Warning: May be habit forming. FOR IV OR IM USE.
PROTECT FROM LIGHT.
Hospira, Inc., Lake Forest, IL 60045 USA   Hospira
```

a. Generic name _____

b. Dosage strength _____

c. Form of the drug _____

d. Routes of administration _____

e. Controlled substance?   yes_____   no_____

f. Multidose _____   Single-dose_____

g. Ordered: 75 mcg IV.
   The nurse will give _____

3.

```
FOR ADMINISTRATION, DILUTE           08917240   NDC 0085-1763-03
with 100 to 200 mLs of suitable diluent.
For complete product information, including Dosage    CIPRO® I.V.
and Administration, see accompanying package
insert.                                            (ciprofloxacin)
INACTIVE INGREDIENTS: Lactic acid as solubilizer,
HCl to adjust pH and Water for Injection, USP.    SINGLE DOSE VIAL contains:
Store between 41-86°F (5-30°C).                    20 mL sterile 1% solution
Protect from light. Avoid freezing.
Manufactured for:                                 200 mg  ciprofloxacin
Bayer Pharmaceuticals Corporation
West Haven, CT 06516                              DILUTE BEFORE USE.
                                                  For Intravenous (iv) Infusion
Distributed by:
Schering Corporation
Kenilworth, NJ 07033                              ℞ Only
CIPRO is a registered trademark of Bayer
Aktiengesellschaft and is used under license                NDC 0085-1763-03
by Schering Corporation.
```

a. Trade name _____

b. Generic name _____

c. Instructions for mixing _____

4.

10 mL Single-dose Preservative-Free **MORPHINE** C Ⅱ **SULFATE** Inj., USP *WARNING: MAY BE HABIT* *FORMING* 5 mg/10 mL (0.5 mg/mL) For I.V., Epidural or Intrathecal Administration. *HOSPIRA, INC., LAKE FOREST, IL 60045 USA*	NDC 0409-4057-12 Each mL contains morphine sulfate, pentahydrate 0.5 mg (Warning: may be habit forming); sodium chloride 9 mg. May contain HCl and/or NaOH for pH adjustment. pH 5.0 (2.5 to 6.5). Store at 20 to 25°C (68 to 77° F). Protect from light. **Do not heat-sterilize.** Do not use if discolored. See insert for dosage and administration. Hospira ℞ only RL-0751 (11/04)

a. Generic name _____

b. Dosage strength _____

c. Total quantity _____

d. Routes of administration _____

e. Controlled substance?   yes ____   no ____

f. Single-dose vial?   yes ____   no ____

g. Ordered: Morphine sulfate 3 mg IV.

   The nurse will give _____

5.

AUGMENTIN® 250mg/5mL **Directions for mixing:** Tap bottle until all powder flows freely. Add approximately 2/3 of total water for reconstitution (total = 87 mL); shake vigorously to wet powder. Add remaining water; again shake vigorously. **Dosage:** See accompanying prescribing information. *Keep tightly closed.* *Shake well before using.* *Must be refrigerated.* *Discard after 10 days*	**250mg/5mL** NDC 0029-6090-23 **AUGMENTIN®** **AMOXICILLIN/** **CLAVULANATE** **POTASSIUM** *FOR ORAL SUSPENSION* When reconstituted, each 5 mL contains: **AMOXICILLIN, 250 MG,** as the trihydrate **CLAVULANIC ACID, 62.5 MG,** as clavulanate potassium **100mL** *(when reconstituted)* GlaxoSmithKline ℞ only

Ordered: Augmentin 375 mg p.o. B.I.D.
   The nurse will give _____

6.

NDC 63323-412-05   410205

MIDAZOLAM HYDROCHLORIDE

INJECTION   (IV)

*25 mg/5 mL

(5 mg/mL)

For IM or IV Use Only

5 mL Vial   Rx only

Sterile
*Each mL contains:
midazolam hydrochloride
equivalent to 5 mg midazolam
compounded with 0.8% sodium
chloride, 0.01% edetate
disodium, with 1% benzyl alcohol
as preservative and pH adjusted
to 3 to 3.6 with hydrochloric acid
and, if necessary, sodium hydroxide.
USUAL DOSAGE: See insert.
Store at controlled room temperature
15° to 30°C (59° to 86°F).
Vial stoppers do not contain natural
rubber latex.

American Pharmaceutical Partners, Inc.
Schaumburg, IL 60173

401852D

LOT

EXP   SAMPL

a. **Generic name** _____

b. **Dosage strength** _____

c. **Routes of administration** _____

d. **Controlled substance?**   yes _____   no _____

e. **Single-dose vial?**   yes _____   no _____

f. **Ordered: Midazolam HCl 12.5 mg IM.**

   The nurse will give _____

7.

LOT / EXP   •   816416504

Rx only
See package insert for
complete product information.
Store at controlled room
temperature 20° to 25°C
(68° to 77°F) [see USPI].
Each mL contains:
Ibutilide fumarate, 0.1 mg;
sodium chloride, 8.90 mg;
sodium acetate trihydrate,
0.189 mg; water for injection.
When necessary, pH was
adjusted with sodium hydroxide
and/or hydrochloric acid.
Pharmacia & Upjohn Company
A subsidiary of
Pharmacia Corporation
Kalamazoo, MI 49001, USA

NDC 0009-3794-01
10 mL

Corvert®

ibutilide fumarate
injection

1 mg/10 mL
(0.1 mg/mL)

Single-Dose Vial
For IV use only

a. **Trade name** _____

b. **Dosage strength** _____

c. **Routes of administration** _____

d. **Storage information** _____

8.

ENALAPRILAT INJECTION	NDC 55390-010-10

ENALAPRILAT
INJECTION

FOR IV USE ONLY

1.25 mg/mL

(Anhydrous equivalent)

NDC 55390-010-10
1 mL Single dose vial
Usual Dosage: See package insert.
Store below 30°C (86°F).
Rx ONLY
Manufactured for:
Bedford Labs™
Bedford, OH 44146   **ENL-V01**

a. Dosage strength _____

b. Routes of administration _____

c. Controlled substance?   yes ____   no ____

d. Ordered: Enalaprilat 0.625 mg IV.

   The nurse will give _____

9.

LEVOTHYROXINE
SODIUM FOR INJECTION

FOR IM OR IV USE ONLY

200 mcg

LYOPHILIZED

Rx ONLY

NDC 55390-880-10
Usual Dosage: See insert for complete information.
Vial contains 200 mcg levothyroxine sodium, 10 mg mannitol, 0.7 mg tribasic sodium phosphate, and sodium hydroxide for pH adjustment.
Use immediately after reconstitution with 5 mL of 0.9% sodium chloride injection, USP only.
Reconstituted concentration is 40 mcg/mL.
Preservative free. Discard any unused portion.
Store at controlled room temperature, 15° to 30°C (59° to 86°F).
Manufactured for:
Bedford Laboratories™
Bedford, OH 44146   **LTR-V04**

a. Dosage strength _____

10.

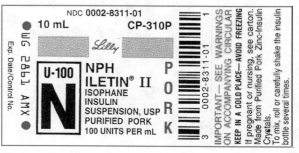

NDC 0002-8311-01
10 mL   CP-310P
Lilly
U-100   NPH   P
N   ILETIN® II   O
      ISOPHANE   R
      INSULIN   K
      SUSPENSION, USP
      PURIFIED PORK
      100 UNITS PER mL

Exp. Date/Control No.

IMPORTANT— SEE WARNINGS ON ACCOMPANYING CIRCULAR
KEEP IN A COLD PLACE— AVOID FREEZING
If pregnant or nursing, see carton.
Made from Purified Pork Zinc-Insulin Crystals.
To mix, roll or carefully shake the insulin bottle several times.

a. Trade name _____

b. Insulin source _____

11.

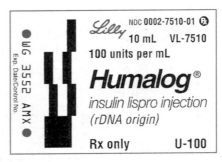

a. Trade name _____

b. Ordered: Humalog 6 units subcut now.
   The nurse will give _____

12.

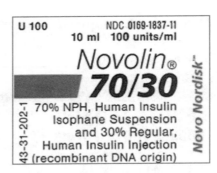

a. Trade name _____

b. Ordered: Novolin 70/30, 22 units subcut now.
   The nurse will give _____

13.

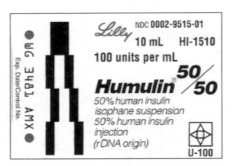

a. Trade name _____

b. Ordered: Humulin 50/50, 17 units subcut q.AM.
   The nurse will give _____

Exercise: FOCUS ON SAFETY

Making Clinical Judgments in Working With Reading Medication Labels

- Read each situation, and then make a clinical judgment.
- Provide a rationale for your decision or action.

SITUATION:
The nurse has an order to administer morphine 3 mg IV stat. The nurse selects the following prefilled syringe. In preparing to administer the ordered dose, it is most important for the nurse to:

a. give 1.5 mL of the prefilled syringe.	c. research the appropriate route of administration.
b. call the pharmacist to double check the order.	d. not administer this drug.

Rationale / Discussion: _____

_____

_____

_____

_____

_____

Module: ORAL MEDICATIONS

ORAL MEDICATIONS

KEY POINTS:
- In setting up oral medication problems, be sure that the units in the medication order and the available drug match.
- Use a conversion table to convert unlike units of measurement.
- When you arrive at the answer, ask yourself if the answer is realistic. Nurses generally administer only 1 – 2 tablets, and less than 30 mL of medication, per dose.

Working With Oral Medications
Solve the following problems using the method of your choice.

1. The physician prescribed 0.8 mg of folic acid q.AM. The pharmacy sends 0.4 mg tablets. How many tablets will the nurse give?

   _____

2. Lanoxin® 0.125 mg is ordered stat. The pharmacy sends 0.25 mg tablets of Lanoxin. How many tablets will the nurse administer?

   _____

3. Levothyroxine 0.1 mg is ordered daily. The pharmacy sends 50 mcg tablets. How many tablets will the nurse give?

   _____

4. The doctor orders acarbose 50 mg p.o. for a patient. How many tablets will the nurse give?

_____

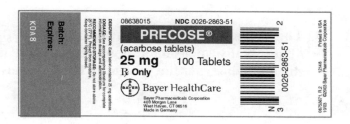

5. The order is for Dilantin® 0.1 g p.o. daily. How many tablets will the nurse give to the patient?

_____

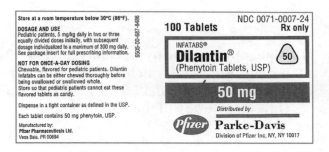

6. Aluminum hydroxide suspension 15 mL is ordered q.i.d. The pharmacy sends a bottle of aluminum hydroxide labeled 320 mg / 5 mL. How many mg is the patient receiving per dose?

_____

7. The patient receives furosemide 80 mg p.o. b.i.d. The pharmacy sends furosemide oral solution labeled 10 mg / mL. How many mL will the nurse give per dose?

_____

8. The nurse is instructing a patient to take Diflucan® 40 mg oral suspension at home. How many tsp will the nurse instruct the patient to take per dose?

_____

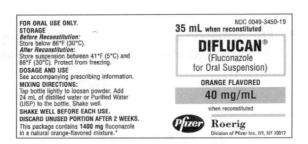

9. Diphenhydramine hydrochloride elixir 50 mg p.o. p.r.n. is ordered for itching. Diphenhydramine hydrochloride elixir 12.5 mg / 5 mL is available. How many mL will the nurse give?

_____

10. The order is for atropine 400 mcg tab i p.o. 30 minutes before surgery. The pharmacy sends atropine 0. 4 mg tablets. How many tablets will the nurse give?

_____

11. The nurse practitioner orders nystatin 200,000 units p.o. q.i.d. p.o., swish and swallow. The pharmacy sends nystatin 100,000 units / 5 mL. How many mL will the nurse give?

_____

12. Nitroglycerin extended-release tablets 5 mg is ordered q.12h. p.o. The pharmacy sends nitroglycerin tablets labeled 2.5 mg / tablet. How many tablets will the nurse give?

_____

13. Augmentin® oral suspension 250 mg q.6h. is ordered for a patient upon discharge. The pharmacy sends the following bottle. How many days will this bottle last?

_____

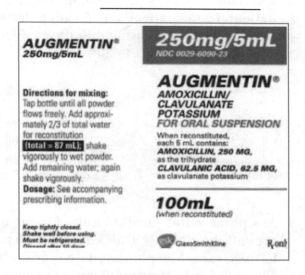

14. The doctor orders enalapril 0.0025 gram p.o. daily. Enalapril is available in 5 mg scored tablets. How many tablets will the nurse give?

_____

15. The order is for cyanocobalamin 1 mg p.o daily. The pharmacy sends cyanocobalamin 1000 mcg tablets. How many tablets will the nurse give?

_____

16. The patient is to receive 20 mEq of KCl p.o. q.AM. The pharmacy sends a bottle labeled 30 mEq / 15 mL. How many mL will the nurse administer?

_____

17. Erythromycin oral suspension 500 mg q.6h. is ordered for a patient. Erythromycin is available in 200 mg / 5 mL. How many mL will the nurse administer?

_____

18. Carvedilol 12.5 mg p.o. b.i.d. is ordered for the patient. In the patient's medication drawer, the nurse finds the following unit dose tablets. The nurse is most correct to administer:

_____

Carvedilol 3.125 mg	Carvedilol 6.25 mg
(4 tablets available)	(2 tablets available)

19. Morphine sulfate oral solution, 120 mg q.4h. around the clock, is ordered for a patient in hospice care. Morphine sulfate is available in 100 mg / 5 mL. How many mg of morphine sulfate will the patient receive per day?

_____

20. Ceclor® oral suspension 375 mg q.8h. is ordered for a patient on discharge. The patient has a prescription for Ceclor 125 mg / 5 mL oral suspension. How many tablespoons will the nurse instruct the patient to take per dose?

_____

21. Mirapex® 1500 mg is ordered t.i.d. for a patient. The nurse has Mirapex 0.5 g tablets. How many tablets will the nurse administer for the morning dose?

_____

22. The patient has an order for levetiracetam oral solution 3 g daily. The patient has a bottle of levetiracetam oral solution 100 mg / mL. How many mL will the nurse administer to the patient?

_____

23. The doctor orders furosemide 40 mg oral solution p.o. q.AM. Furosemide 8 mg / mL oral solution is available. The nurse has a medicine cup with ounce measurements. How many ounces will the nurse administer to the patient?

_____

24. The nurse is preparing to administer the 0900 medications to a patient. In the medication drawer, the nurse finds the following unit dose tablets: digoxin 0.25 mg scored tablet, Captopril® 12.5 mg tablet, furosemide 10 mg tablets, Cipro® 500 mg tablets. How many tablets of each of the medications will the nurse administer at 0900?

Digoxin 0.125 mg p.o. q.AM	0900
Captopril 12.5 mg p.o. q.12h.	0900 2100
Furosemide 20 mg p.o. B.I.D.	0900 1700
Cipro 0.5 g p.o. q.12h.	0800 2000

_____

Exercise: FOCUS ON SAFETY
Making Clinical Judgments in Working With Oral Medications

- Read each situation, and then make a clinical judgment.
- Provide a rationale for your decision or action.

Hydralazine 25 mg p.o. Q.I.D	0900 - 1300 1800 2200	K-Dur 8 mEq
K-Dur 16 mEq p.o. T.I.D.	0900 - 1300 2100	K-Dur 8 mEq
Propranolol 60 mg p.o. B.I.D.	0900 - 1700	Propranolol 60 mg ER
		Hydralazine 25 mg

SITUATION:
The nurse is preparing the 0900 medications and finds the patient's unit dose medications in the medication drawer. Which action(s) by the nurse are most appropriate (select all that apply)?

a. Give all the 0900 medications.

b. Call the pharmacist regarding the propranolol.

c. Call the pharmacist regarding the K-Dur®.

d. Give the hydralazine and the K-Dur at 0900.

e. Give the hydralazine and propranolol at 0900.

Rationale / Discussion:

Module: SYRINGES AND NEEDLES

SYRINGES

KEY POINTS:
- The most commonly used syringe, the 3 mL syringe, is calibrated to measure 0.1 mL accurately. Most 3 mL syringes have both minim and mL scales.
- The TB syringe measures volumes of 1 mL or less, and is calibrated to measure 0.01 mL accurately. The TB syringe has minim and mL scales.
- Larger volume syringes are calibrated in 0.2 mL or 1 mL increments.
- Insulin is measured in units and is drawn up in an insulin syringe. The standard insulin syringe is calibrated by 2 unit increments. Low dosage insulin syringes are calibrated in 1 unit increments.

Working With Syringes
Shade in the syringe with the indicated amount of medication.

1. 0.3 mL

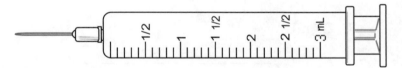

2. 0.66 mL

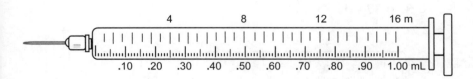

3. 0.09 mL

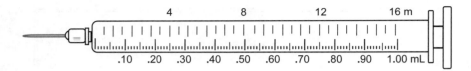

4. 7.5 minims

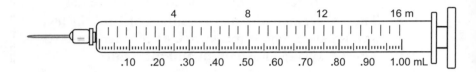

5. 15 minims

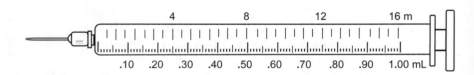

6. 1.2 mL

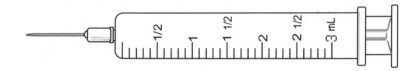

7. 2.7 mL

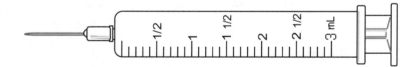

8. 0.37 mL

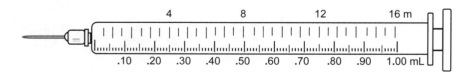

9. 1.9 mL

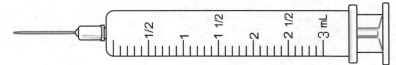

10. 4.6 mL

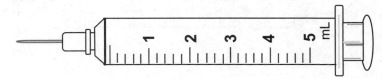

11. 38 units

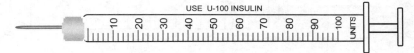

12. 27 units

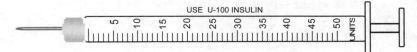

13. 7 units

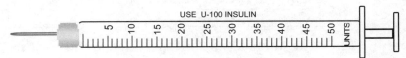

14. 7 units

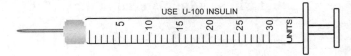

15. 16 units

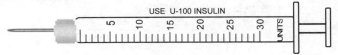

16.   56 units

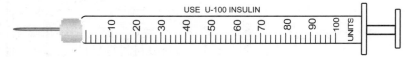

17.   72 units

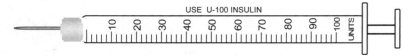

18.   3.8 mL

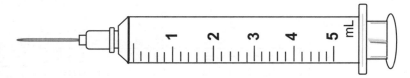

19.   The nurse has a 1 mL prefilled syringe with digoxin 250 mcg / mL. The nurse has an order for 0.125 mg IV. Shade in the amount of digoxin that will be administered to the patient.

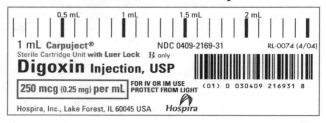

20.   The nurse has a 2 mL prefilled syringe with fentanyl 100 mcg / 2 mL The nurse has an order for 75 mcg IV. Shade in the amount of fentanyl that will be administered to the patient.

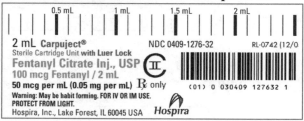

Exercise: FOCUS ON SAFETY
Making Clinical Judgments in Working With Syringes

- Read each situation, and then make a clinical judgment.
- Provide a rationale for your decision or action.

SITUATION:
After calculating the ordered dose of a medication, the nurse determines that the patient is to receive 5 mL of the medication IM. The nurse selects a 5 mL syringe to administer the ordered dose. The nurse:

a. has correctly determined the most appropriate syringe to measure and administer this dose accurately.

b. needs to contact the physician and request a higher dosage strength of the medication.

c. needs to contact the pharmacist to ensure that the ordered dose has been correctly calculated.

d. should divide the medication into two injections, using two 3 mL syringes.

Rationale / Discussion:

NEEDLES

KEY POINTS:
- Needles are identified by two numbers: length and gauge.
- Needle length is measured in inches.
- Needle gauge refers to the diameter. The larger the number of the gauge, the smaller the diameter of the needle.
- Needles are packaged in standard sizes with syringes for IM, ID, subcut, and IV use.

Working With Needles
Choose the correct needle size for the following injections.

1. A subcut injection of insulin   _____

2. An IM injection   _____

3. A TB skin test   _____

4. An IM injection for an obese person

    _____

5. A subcut injection into the upper arm

    _____

6. Drawing up viscous medication from a vial

    _____

Choose the correct syringe and needle for the following injections. Fill in the syringe.

1. Meperidine 75 mg (1 mL) IM

a.

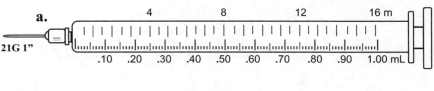

21G 1"

b.

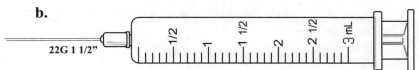

22G 1 1/2"

2. Filgrastim 300 mcg (1 mL) subcut

a.

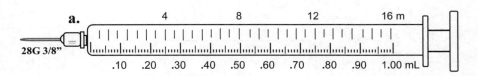

28G 3/8"

b.

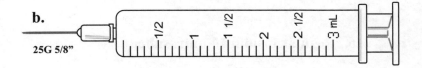

25G 5/8"

3. Heparin 5000 units (0.67 mL) subcut

a.

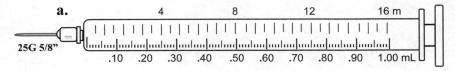

25G 5/8"

b.

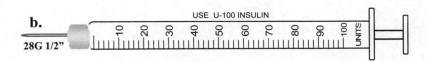

28G 1/2"

4. Hepatitis A vaccine 1 mL IM

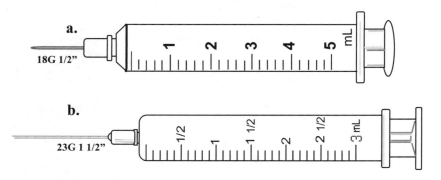

5. Ketorolac 60 mg (2 mL) IM

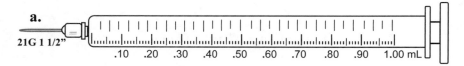

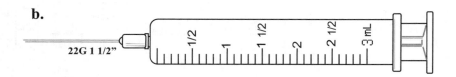

6. Regular insulin 17 units subcut

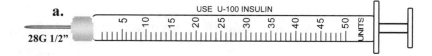

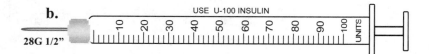

7. Regular insulin 6 units and NPH insulin 13 units subcut

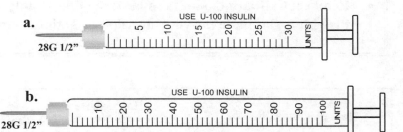

8. Heparin 1000 units (0.1 mL) subcut

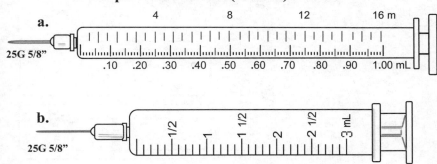

9. Morphine sulfate 10 mg (16 minims) subcut

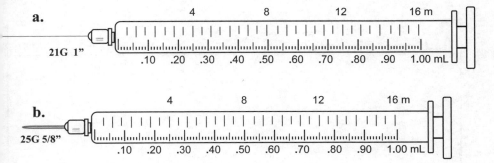

Exercise: FOCUS ON SAFETY
Making Clinical Judgments in Working With Needles

- Read each situation, and then make a clinical judgment.
- Provide a rationale for your decision or action.

Date	Medication Record	
7/29	Heparin 5,000 units subcut into the abdomen q.AM	0900
	Patient T	

SITUATION:
To administer this medication safely, it is most correct for the nurse to use a:

a. 18G 1"

b. 20G 1 1/2"

c. 22G 1"

d. 25G 1/2"

Rationale / Discussion:

Module: PARENTERAL MEDICATIONS

PARENTERAL MEDICATIONS

KEY POINTS:

- In setting up parenteral medication problems, be sure that the units in the medication order and the available drug are the same.
- Use a conversion table to convert unlike units of measurement.
- When you arrive at the answer, ask yourself if the answer is realistic. Nurses generally administer 3 mL or less of a parenteral medication.
- With insulin, just draw up the total units ordered.

Working With Parenteral Medications
Use of method of your choice to solve the problems.

1. The physician prescribed 0.1 mg of folic acid IM. The pharmacy sends the following ampule. How many mL will the nurse give?

   _____

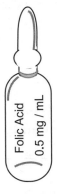

Folic Acid
0.5 mg / mL

2. Meperidine HCl 75 mg is ordered stat. Meperidine HCl 50 mg / mL is available. How many mL will the nurse administer?

   _____

3. Heparin sodium 5,000 units subcut q.12h. is ordered for a patient. The pharmacy sends a vial labeled heparin sodium 20,000 units / mL. How many mL will the nurse give?

_____

4. Procaine penicillin G 1.2 million units IM is ordered for a patient. The pharmacy sends procaine penicillin G 600,000 units / mL. How many mL will the nurse give?

_____

Fill in the syringe.

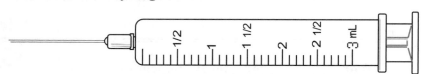

5. The preoperative order is morphine sulfate 9 mg with glycopyrrolate 0.08 mg IM stat. Morphine sulfate 15 mg / mL and glycopyrrolate 200 mcg / mL are available in the medication drawer. Calculate the preoperative medications.

Morphine sulfate: _____

Glycopyrrolate: _____

Fill in the syringe with the total amount.

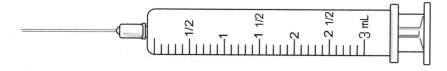

6. Hydromorphone 1 mg subcut q.3h. p.r.n. for pain is ordered for a patient. Hydromorphone 10 mg / mL is available in the narcotic drawer. How many mL will the nurse give?

_____

Fill in the ordered dose in each syringe.

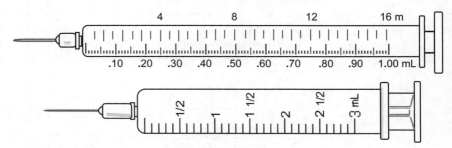

7. The order is for atropine 400 mcg subcut now. The pharmacy sends the following multidose vial. How many mL will the nurse give?

_____

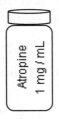

Atropine
1 mg / mL

8. The physician orders morphine sulfate 0.015 gram. Morphine sulfate is available in 15 mg / mL. How many minims will the nurse give?

_____

Fill in the syringe.

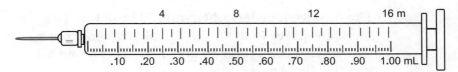

9. **Epoetin 12,000 units subcut 3x / week is ordered. The pharmacy sends a vial of epoetin labeled 20,000 units / mL. How many mL will the nurse give?**

_____

Fill in the ordered dose in each syringe.

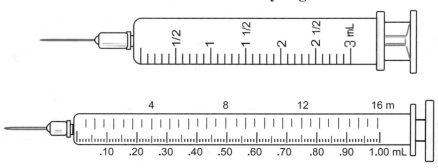

10. **The doctor orders ampicillin 250 mg. The pharmacy sends a vial of ampicillin labeled 1 g / mL. How many mL will the nurse give?**

_____

Fill in the ordered dose in the most appropriate syringe.

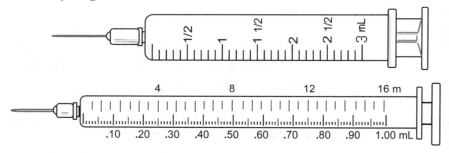

11. **The physician orders phenytoin 125 mg IM. The nurse prepares to draw up the medication from a vial labeled phenytoin 50 mg / mL. How many mL will the nurse give?**

_____

12. **Humulin NPH insulin 23 units q.AM is ordered for a patient. How much insulin will the nurse give?**

Fill in the most appropriate syringe.

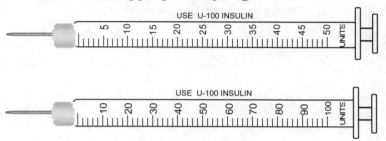

13. **Humulin Lente insulin 35 units and Humulin Regular insulin 17 units q.AM are ordered for a patient. How much insulin will the nurse give?**

Fill in the most appropriate syringe.

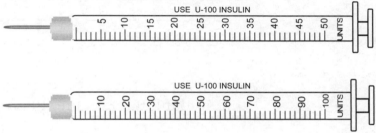

14. **Humulin 70/30 insulin 21 units q.AM is ordered for the patient. How much insulin will the nurse give?**

Fill in the most appropriate syringe.

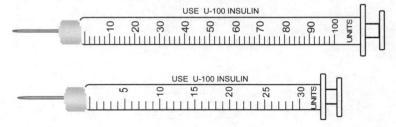

15. Humulin 50/50 insulin 19 units q.AM is ordered for the patient. How much insulin will the nurse give?

Fill in the most appropriate syringe.

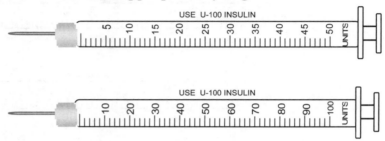

16. Humulin Regular insulin 2 units is ordered for the patient. How much insulin will the nurse give?

Fill in the most appropriate syringe.

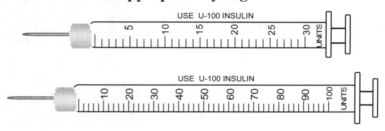

17. Humulin NPH insulin 22 units and Humulin Regular insulin 7 units are ordered stat. How much insulin will the nurse give?

Fill in the most appropriate syringe.

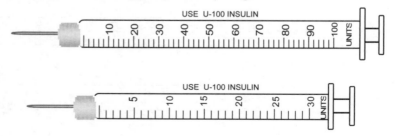

18. Adenosine 2.7 mg IV is ordered. The pharmacy sends a 2 mL single-dose vial of adenosine. How many mL will the nurse administer?

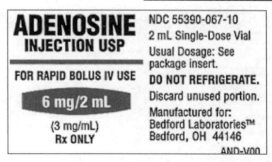

19. Midazolam HCl 6 mg IV is ordered. The nurse has the following vial of midazolam HCl. How many mL will the nurse administer?

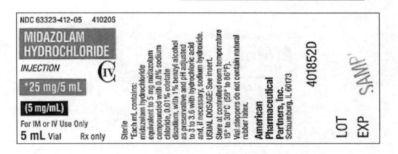

20. The nurse receives an order to administer ranitidine 20 mg IVP. How many mL will the nurse administer?

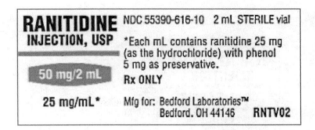

21. **Propranolol HCL 500 mcg is ordered IVP. To carry out this order correctly, the nurse will administer how many mL of propranolol HCl?**

_____

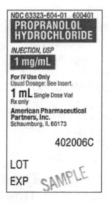

22. **The physician orders amikacin 0.25 g IM q.12h. How many mL will the nurse administer per dose?**

_____

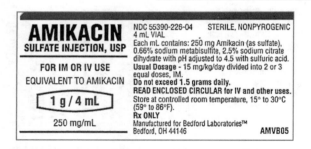

23. **Enalaprilat 0.625 mg IVP q.6h. is ordered. After drawing up the ordered dose, how many mL will the nurse discard from the vial?**

_____

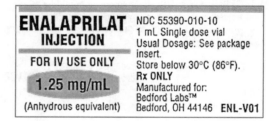

Exercise: FOCUS ON SAFETY
Making Clinical Judgments in Working With Parenteral Medications

- Read each situation, and then make a clinical judgment.
- Provide a rationale for your decision or action.

SITUATION:
The nurse has an order to administer levothyroxine 0.065 mg IVP q.AM. How many mL will the nurse draw into the syringe?

LEVOTHYROXINE SODIUM FOR INJECTION

FOR IM OR IV USE ONLY

200 mcg

LYOPHILIZED

Rx ONLY

NDC 55390-880-10
Usual Dosage: See insert for complete information.
Vial contains 200 mcg levothyroxine sodium, 10 mg mannitol, 0.7 mg tribasic sodium phosphate, and sodium hydroxide for pH adjustment.
Use immediately after reconstitution with 5 mL of 0.9% sodium chloride injection, USP only. Reconstituted concentration is 40 mcg/mL. Preservative free. Discard any unused portion.
Store at controlled room temperature, 15° to 30°C (59° to 86°F).
Manufactured for:
Bedford Laboratories™
Bedford, OH 44146   LTR-V04

a. 0.33 mL

c. 1.5 mL

b. 1.38 mL

d. 1.63 mL

Rationale / Discussion:

Module: RECONSTITUTION OF POWDERED MEDICATIONS

SINGLE-STRENGTH RECONSTITUTION

KEY POINTS:
- In single-strength reconstitution, the manufacturer identifies one amount of diluent to add to the powdered medication.
- The dosage strength of the mixed medication is used to calculate the amount to give to the patient.
- Information needed to work with single-strength reconstitution problems includes the type and amount of diluent, dosage strength of the mixed medication, length of time the solution will remain stable, and storage information.
- Once the medication is reconstituted, the nurse writes the date and time of reconstitution and the nurse's initials on the medication label.

Working With Single-Strength Reconstitution
Solve the following single-strength reconstitution problems.

1. The physician orders cefazolin sodium 0.25 g IM q.8h. The pharmacy sends a 1 g vial of sterile cefazolin powder with the following mixing instructions: "For IM use, add 2.5 mL sterile water for injection and shake. Provides a volume of 3.0 mL (330 mg / mL)."

  a. How much diluent will be added to the cefazolin sodium powder?

  _____

b. What type of diluent will be added?

_____

c. What is the dosage strength of the mixed medication?

_____

d. How many mL of the medication will the nurse give to the patient?

_____

2. The order is for procaine penicillin G 300,000 units IM b.i.d. A 1 gram vial of procaine penicillin G powder is in the medication drawer. The medication has the following mixing instructions: "IM use: Dissolve 4.6 mL bacteriostatic water for injection to make 200,000 units / mL."

a. How much diluent will be added to the procaine penicillin G powder?

_____

b. What type of diluent will be added?

_____

c. What is the dosage strength of the mixed medication?

_____

d. How many mL of the medication will the nurse give to the patient?

_____

3. What data should be entered on the vial below when labeling the vial after reconstitution?

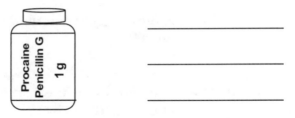

Procaine Penicillin G
1 g

_____

_____

_____

4. The physician orders 200 mg of an antibiotic IM q.12h. The pharmacy sends a vial of antibiotic powder for reconstitution with the following mixing directions: "For IM injection, IV direct (bolus) injection, or IV infusion, add 2 mL sterile water for injection. Shake well. Provides an approximate concentration of 125 mg / mL."

a. How much diluent will be added to the antibiotic powder?

_____

b. What type of diluent will be added?

_____

c. What is the dosage strength of the mixed medication?

_____

d. How many mL of the medication will the nurse give to the patient?

_____

5. The order is for ticarcillin disodium 0.5 g IM q.6h. The directions state to add 2 mL of NS. The reconstituted solution contains 1 g / 2.6 mL.

   a. What is the dosage strength of the reconstituted medication?

   _____

   b. How much will be given to the patient?

   _____

6. The order is for cefazolin 450 mg IM q.6h.

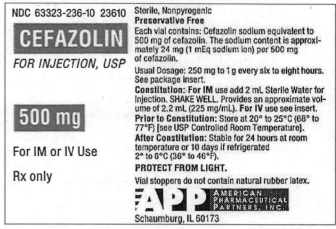

NDC 63323-236-10 23610

CEFAZOLIN

FOR INJECTION, USP

500 mg

For IM or IV Use

Rx only

Sterile, Nonpyrogenic
Preservative Free
Each vial contains: Cefazolin sodium equivalent to 500 mg of cefazolin. The sodium content is approximately 24 mg (1 mEq sodium ion) per 500 mg of cefazolin.
Usual Dosage: 250 mg to 1 g every six to eight hours. See package insert.
Constitution: For IM use add 2 mL Sterile Water for Injection. SHAKE WELL. Provides an approximate volume of 2.2 mL (225 mg/mL). For IV use see insert.
Prior to Constitution: Store at 20° to 25°C (68° to 77°F) [see USP Controlled Room Temperature].
After Constitution: Stable for 24 hours at room temperature or 10 days if refrigerated 2° to 8°C (36° to 46°F).
PROTECT FROM LIGHT.
Vial stoppers do not contain natural rubber latex.
APP AMERICAN PHARMACEUTICAL PARTNERS, INC.
Schaumburg, IL 60173

   a. How much diluent will be added to the cefazolin powder?

   _____

   b. What type of diluent will be added?

   _____

   c. What is the resulting dosage strength of the mixed medication?

   _____

   d. How many mL of the cefazolin will the nurse give to the patient?

   _____

7. **The physician orders Augmentin ® 500 mg p.o. q.12h. The pharmacy sends the following drug:**

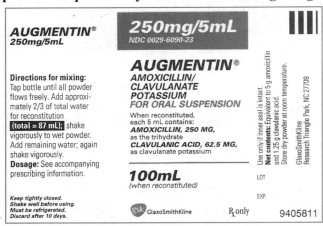

a. How much diluent will be added to the Augmentin powder?

_____

b. What is the dosage strength of the mixed medication?

_____

c. How many mL of the Augmentin oral suspension will the nurse give to the patient?

_____

d. What data should be entered on the label above after reconstitution?

_____

_____

_____

8. **The order is for 0.5 g IV of a drug. Reconstitution instructions for the powdered medication include: "Reconstitute with 2 mL bacteriostatic water (with benzyl alcohol) for injection. Resulting dosage strength is 300 mg / mL." How many mL will the nurse give?**

_____

Exercise: FOCUS ON SAFETY
Making Clinical Judgments in Working With
Single-Strength Reconstitution

- Read each situation, and then make a clinical judgment.
- Provide a rationale for your decision or action.

AUGMENTIN®
250mg/5mL

250mg/5mL
NDC 0029-6090-23

‖‖‖

AUGMENTIN®
AMOXICILLIN/
CLAVULANATE
POTASSIUM
FOR ORAL SUSPENSION

Directions for mixing:
Tap bottle until all powder flows freely. Add approximately 2/3 of total water for reconstitution **(total = 87 mL);** shake vigorously to wet powder. Add remaining water; again shake vigorously.
Dosage: See accompanying prescribing information.

When reconstituted, each 5 mL contains:
AMOXICILLIN, 250 MG,
as the trihydrate
CLAVULANIC ACID, 62.5 MG,
as clavulanate potassium

Use only if inner seal is intact. **Net contents:** Equivalent to 5 g amoxicillin and 1.25 g clavulanic acid. Store dry powder at room temperature.

GlaxoSmithKline
Research Triangle Park, NC 27709

100mL
(when reconstituted)

JC RN
1500

LOT
EXP.

Keep tightly closed.
Shake well before using.
Must be refrigerated.
Discard after 10 days.

gsk GlaxoSmithKline

℞only

9405811

SITUATION:
The nurse has an order to administer 250 mg of Augmentin. The nurse measures 1 tsp. Which action by the nurse is most correct?

a. Convert the tsp to mL.

c. Question the date of reconstitution.

b. Administer the measured dose.

d. Use a 3 mL syringe to measure the dose.

Rationale / Discussion:

_____

_____

_____

_____

_____

_____

MULTIPLE-STRENGTH RECONSTITUTION

KEY POINTS:
- In multiple-strength reconstitution, the manufacturer identifies several amounts of diluent to add to the powdered medication.
- The nurse must select one of the listed amounts of diluent.
- The dosage strength of the mixed medication is used to calculate the amount to give to the patient.
- Information needed to work with multiple-strength reconstitution problems includes the type and amount of diluent, dosage strength of the mixed medication, length of time the solution will remain stable, and storage information.
- Once the medication is reconstituted, the nurse circles the amount of diluent selected and the corresponding dosage strength. The date and time of reconstitution and the nurse's initials are also written on the medication label.

Working With Multiple-Strength Reconstitution
Solve the following multiple-strength reconstitution problems.

1. When preparing multiple-strength reconstitution medications, the nurse will make the most concentrated solution when adding:

☐ the largest volume of diluent.

☐ the smallest volume of diluent.

2. The physician orders cefoperazone 750 mg IV q.12h. The pharmacy sends a 2 g vial of sterile cefoperazone powder with the following mixing instructions: "Diluent: sterile bacteriostatic water for injection. Add 10 mL for an approximate volume of 100 mg / mL. Add 15 mL for an approximate volume of 150 mg / mL."

   a. What is the dosage strength if the nurse chooses to add 10 mL of diluent?

   _____

   b. How many mL of the mixed solution will the nurse administer to the patient?

   _____

   c. What information should be written on the label of the reconstituted cefoperazone?

   _____
   _____
   _____
   _____

3. The physician orders penicillin G potassium 1 million units IV q.6h. The nurse has a vial with the following instructions:

Add Diluent (mL)	Dosage Strength of Mixed Medication
9.6	100,000 units / mL
4.6	200,000 units / mL
1.6	500,000 units / mL

   a. What is the dosage strength if the nurse chooses to add 9.6 mL of diluent?

   _____

b. What is the dosage strength if the nurse chooses to add 1.6 mL of diluent?

_____

c. Select one volume of diluent, and calculate the amount of penicillin G potassium to administer.

_____

4. The physician orders 750,000 units of penicillin G potassium. The nurse has the following vial:

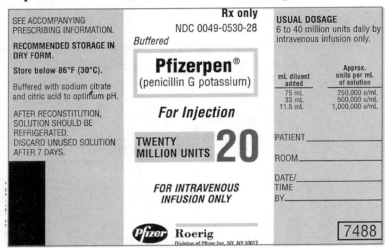

a. Select one volume of diluent. What is the dosage strength of the mixed medication if this volume of diluent is added to the vial?

_____

b. Calculate the amount of medication to administer.

_____

c. How long is the solution stable if refrigerated?

_____

d. Complete the label with the correct information.

5. The physician orders ampicillin 700 mg IV q.6h. The nurse has a vial of powdered ampicillin with the following directions for reconstitution:

For IM or IV use: Add bacteriostatic NS or sterile water for injection and shake.

Diluent	Strength of Mixed Medication
3.5 mL	500 mg / mL
7.2 mL	250 mg / mL

Use within 1 hour of reconstitution. Stable under refrigeration for 6 hours. See package insert.

a. Select one volume of diluent. What is the dosage strength of the mixed medication if this volume of diluent is added to the vial?

_____

b. Calculate the amount of medication to administer.

_____

c. How long is the mixed solution stable?

_____

d. If the ampicillin is given IM, which diluent volume would be preferable? Why?

_____

e. Complete the label with the appropriate information.

6. The physician orders Ancef ® 500 mg IM q.8h. The nurse has a vial of powdered Ancef with the following directions:

equivalent to
1gram cefazolin
NDC 0007-3130-01
ANCEF®
CEFAZOLIN FOR
INJECTION
(LYOPHILIZED)
For I.V. or I.M. use
EXP.
LOT
R only
gsk GlaxoSmithKline

Before reconstitution protect from light and store at Controlled Room Temperature 20° to 25°C (68° to 77°F).
Each vial contains cefazolin sodium equivalent to 1 gram of cefazolin. The sodium content is 48 mg per gram of cefazolin.
Usual Adult Dosage: 250 mg to 1 gram every 6 to 8 hours. See accompanying prescribing information. Reconstituted *Ancef* is stable 24 hours at room temperature or 10 days if refrigerated (5°C or 41°F).
GlaxoSmithKline
Research Triangle Park, NC 27709   693820-AA

a. After reading the label, the nurse can identify the (check all that apply):

☐ routes of administration

☐ storage information

☐ dosage strength

☐ usual adult dosage

☐ type of diluent

b. To administer the ordered dose (500 mg) the nurse:

☐ needs to call the pharmacist for mixing instructions.

☐ should read the accompanying literature.

☐ will give 2 mL of the reconstituted drug.

Exercise: FOCUS ON SAFETY
Making Clinical Judgments in Working With Multiple-Strength Reconstitution

- Read each situation, and then make a clinical judgment.
- Provide a rationale for your decision or action.

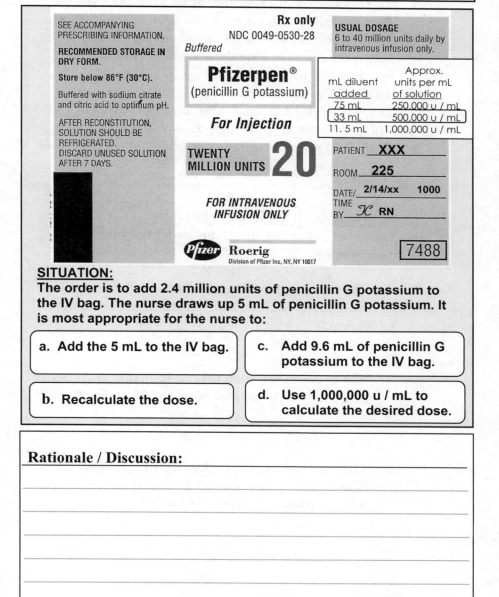

SEE ACCOMPANYING PRESCRIBING INFORMATION.

RECOMMENDED STORAGE IN DRY FORM.

Store below 86°F (30°C).

Buffered with sodium citrate and citric acid to optimum pH.

AFTER RECONSTITUTION, SOLUTION SHOULD BE REFRIGERATED. DISCARD UNUSED SOLUTION AFTER 7 DAYS.

Rx only
NDC 0049-0530-28
Buffered

Pfizerpen®
(penicillin G potassium)

For Injection

TWENTY MILLION UNITS **20**

FOR INTRAVENOUS INFUSION ONLY

Pfizer Roerig
Division of Pfizer Inc, NY, NY 10017

USUAL DOSAGE
6 to 40 million units daily by intravenous infusion only.

mL diluent added	Approx. units per mL of solution
75 mL	250,000 u / mL
33 mL	500,000 u / mL
11.5 mL	1,000,000 u / mL

PATIENT **XXX**

ROOM **225**

DATE/ **2/14/xx   1000**
TIME
BY **JC RN**

7488

SITUATION:
The order is to add 2.4 million units of penicillin G potassium to the IV bag. The nurse draws up 5 mL of penicillin G potassium. It is most appropriate for the nurse to:

a. Add the 5 mL to the IV bag.

c. Add 9.6 mL of penicillin G potassium to the IV bag.

b. Recalculate the dose.

d. Use 1,000,000 u / mL to calculate the desired dose.

Rationale / Discussion:

Module: IV CALCULATIONS

Working With Milliliters per Hour
Solve the following problems using the method of your choice.

1. The order is for 1000 mL D5/0.225% NS q.12h. How many mL / hr will the nurse set on the IV pump?

   _____

2. The order is for 1000 mL D5W q.16h. How many mL / hr will the nurse set on the IV pump?

   _____

3. The physician orders 3000 mL of Lactated Ringer's to infuse over 24 hours. How many mL will the patient receive per hour?

   _____

4. The order is to infuse 1 unit of packed red blood cells (250 mL) over 1 ½ hours. Calculate the mL / hr.

    _____

5. The doctor orders ceftizoxime 1 g IVPB q.12h. The pharmacy sends ceftizoxime 1 g in 50 mL NS to infuse over 30 minutes. Calculate the mL / hr.

    _____

6. The physician orders 1 L 0.9% NS to infuse over 6 hours. Calculate the mL / hr.

    _____

7. The order is to infuse 500 mL of D5W over 10 hrs. Calculate the mL / hr.

    _____

8. The order is to infuse 1 unit of packed red blood cells (275 mL) over 2 hours. Calculate the mL / hr.

    _____

9. The physician orders 250 mL 0.9% NS to infuse over 2 ½ hours. Calculate the mL / hr.

    _____

10. The doctor orders vancomycin 1 g IVPB q.12h. The pharmacy sends vancomycin 1 g in 200 mL 0.9% NS to infuse over 90 minutes. Calculate the mL / hr.

    _____

Working With Flow Rate

1. The nurse hangs up 1 L D5W to infuse over 8 hours. Use the following IV tubing label to calculate the flow rate.

    _____

    ┌─────────────────────────────┐
    │ **Primary IV Set**   │
    │ **Non-Vented, 72 inch**   │
    │   │
    │ **60 drops / mL**   │
    └─────────────────────────────┘

2. The physician orders 1 L of D5LR to infuse at 83 mL / hr. The IV tubing delivers 15 gtt / mL. What is the flow rate (gtt / min)?

    _____

3. The doctor orders 1 unit of whole blood (500 mL) to infuse over 4 hours. The blood tubing delivers 10 gtt / mL. What is the flow rate of the blood?

    _____

4. The order is for 500 mL of NS TKO (30 mL / hr). The nurse selects the following IV tubing. What is the flow rate?

    _____

    ┌─────────────────────────────┐
    │ **Primary IV Set**   │
    │ **Non-Vented, 72 inch**   │
    │   │
    │ **15 drops / mL**   │
    └─────────────────────────────┘

5. The IV is to infuse at 42 mL / hr. The drop factor on the IV tubing is 15 gtt / mL. What is the flow rate?

_____

6. The order is to infuse 250 mL of NS over 1 ½ hours. The drop factor is 12 gtt / mL. What is the flow rate?

_____

7. The order is for 500 mL of D5/0.45% NS to infuse over 4 hours. The nurse selects the following IV tubing. What is the flow rate?

_____

```
Primary IV Set
Non-Vented, 72 inch

15 drops / mL
```

8. The nurse is to infuse vancomycin 1 g in 250 mL 0.9% NS over 1 ½ hours. The nurse selects a minidrop tubing (60 gtt / mL). Calculate the flow rate.

_____

9. The patient is to receive 1 unit whole blood (475 mL) to infuse over 3 hours. The nurse starts the transfusion using blood tubing labeled 10 gtt / mL. What is the flow rate?

_____

10. The nurse is to infuse 1 liter D10W over 8 hours. The nurse selects IV tubing label 12 gtt / mL. Calculate the flow rate.

_____

Exercise: FOCUS ON SAFETY
Making Clinical Judgments in Working With Milliliters per Hour and Flow Rate

- Read each situation, and then make a clinical judgment.
- Provide a rationale for your decision or action.

Intake and Output

7 – 3	Oral	IV	Urine	Emesis	Other
	400	350	250		
			200		
			225		
Total mL	400	350	675		
3 – 11					

**Primary IV Set
Non-Vented, 72 inch
15 drops / mL**

SITUATION:
The nurse started an IV of 500 mL NS 0.9% at 0800, to infuse over 10 hours via gravity. The IV infused at 13 gtt /min all shift.

At 1500, the end of the shift, the nurse completed the intake and output record.

In reviewing the Intake and Output record, the nurse from the evening shift is most correct to:

a. continue to monitor the IV at 13 gtt / min.

c. increase the flow rate to 31 gtt / min.

b. question the oral intake for the day shift.

d. change the IV tubing to a minidrop.

Rationale / Discussion:

IV PUSH MEDICATIONS

KEY POINTS:
- Use a drug reference book to find the rate of administration for IV push medications.
- If the dosage ordered is smaller than the recommended dose in the drug reference book, administer the dosage over the full amount of time recommended.
- The term "fraction thereof" in a drug reference book means that any fraction of a dose is given over the full amount of time recommended.

Working With IV Push Medication
Use the information provided to identify the IV push rate of administration for the following problems.

1. The doctor orders morphine sulfate 10 mg IVP stat. The recommended rate of administration is 15 mg or fraction thereof over 4 – 5 minutes. What is the rate of administration for this dose?

   _____

2. The doctor orders hydromorphone 3 mg IV for severe pain. The drug reference literature states "Administer slowly at a rate not to exceed 2 mg over 3 – 5 min. Rapid infusion may lead to respiratory depression, hypotension, and circulatory collapse." What is the rate of administration for this dose?

   _____

3. The doctor orders furosemide 80 mg IVP now. What is the rate of administration for this dose?

_____

---

furosemide
(fur-**oh**-se-mide)

IMPLEMENTATION

- **Direct IV: Administer undiluted.**
  Rate: **Administer slowly over 1 – 2 minutes.**
- **Intermittent Infusion: Dilute large doses.**
  Rate: **Not to exceed 4 mg / min.**

---

4. The doctor orders methylprednisolone sodium succinate 250 mg IVP q.AM. The recommended rate of administration is 500 mg over 2 – 3 minutes or longer. What is the rate of administration for this dose?

_____

5. The doctor orders diazepam 10 mg IVP now. The drug book states "Administer slowly at a rate of 5 mg over at least 1 minute." What is the rate of administration for this dose?

_____

6. The doctor orders lorazepam 0.001 gram IVP 30 minutes before chemotherapy. What is the rate of administration for this dose?

_____

---

lorazepam
(lor-**az**-e-pam)

IMPLEMENTATION

- *Rate:* Administer direct IV, through Y-site at a rate of 2 mg over 1 minute. Rapid IV administration may result in apnea, hypotension, bradycardia, or cardiac arrest.

---

7. The doctor orders phenytoin 75 mg IVP for a patient experiencing status epilepticus. What is the rate of administration for this dose?

_____

---

phenytoin
(**fen**-i-toyn)

IMPLEMENTATION

- Direct IV: Administer at a rate not to exceed 50 mg over 1 minute (25 mg / min [may be as low as 5 – 10 mg / min] in patients who may develop hypotension).

Exercise: FOCUS ON SAFETY
Making Clinical Judgments in Working With IV Push Medication

- Read each situation, and then make a clinical judgment.
- Provide a rationale for your decision or action.

Date	Physician's Orders
2/12	Atropine 0.8 mg IVP stat

Patient C
ID *******

atropine
(at-ro-peen)

IMPLEMENTATION
- Direct IV: Give IV undiluted or dilute in 10 mL sterile water.

- *Rate:* Administer at a rate of 0.6 mg over 1 min. Do not add to solution. Inject through Y- tubing or 3-way stopcock.

SITUATION:
Atropine is available in 1 mg / mL. To implement this order safely, the nurse is most correct to:

a. give the ordered dose slowly into the vein.

c. add the atropine dose to the primary IV fluid.

b. administer 0.8 mL over 2 minutes.

d. Dilute with 10 mL normal saline.

Rationale / Discussion:

86   Copyright © 2007, F. A. Davis Company

INFUSION AND COMPLETION TIME

KEY POINTS:
- Use mL / hr and total amount of IV fluid to calculate the infusion time (hours and minutes).
- Use the starting time and the infusion time to calculate the completion time of the IV fluid.
- With infusion time, convert parts of an hour to minutes.

Working With Infusion Time
Use the information provided to identify the infusion time for the following problems.

1. The doctor orders 1 L of D5/0.45% NS to infuse at 125 mL / hr. What is the infusion time of the IV?

   _____

2. At 0700, 500 mL of D5W is started to infuse at 60 mL / hr. What is the infusion time of the IV?

   _____

3. At 1000, 1000 mL of Lactated Ringer's is started on the patient. The IV is infusing at 75 mL / hr. The drop factor is 10 gtt / min. What is the infusion time of the IV?

   _____

4. The nurse restarts an IV with 800 mL D5/LR to infuse at 125 mL / hr. What is the infusion time of the IV?

   _____

5. The patient has an IVPB of famotidine 20 mg in 100 mL NS. The nurse sets the IV pump at 200 mL / hr. What is the infusion time of the IVPB?

_____

6. The nurse starts an IV of 100 mL D5W with 10 mEq KCl to infuse at 30 mL / hr. What is the infusion time of the IV?

_____

Working With Completion Time

1. The nurse starts 1 L of D5/0.45% NS to infuse at 125 mL / hr at 0800. What is the completion time of this IV?

_____

2. At 1400, 250 mL of D5W is started to infuse at 60 mL / hr. What is the completion time of the IV?

_____

3. At 2000, 1000 mL of 0.45% NS is started to infuse at 100 mL / hr. What is the completion time of the IV?

_____

4. The nurse restarts an IV bag containing 600 mL of IV fluid at 1930 to infuse at 75 mL / hr. What is the completion time of the IV?

_____

5. The nurse restarts an IV bag containing 500 mL of D5/0.45% NS at 1430, to infuse at 80 mL / hr. What is the completion time of this IV?

_____

6. The nurse restarts 750 mL of LR at 0900, to infuse at 150 mL / hr. What is the completion time of the IV?

_____

Working With Infusion and Completion Time

1. The doctor orders 1 L NS to infuse over 10 hours. The nurse starts the IV at 0900. At 1000 the patient pulls out the IV. The nurse restarts the IV at 1100 at the same rate. Starting with the amount of IV fluid left at 1100, calculate the new infusion time and the completion time of the IV.

   Infusion time_____

   Completion time_____

2. The doctor orders 500 mL D10W to infuse at 75 mL / hr. The nurse starts the IV at 1330. At 1530, the IV rate is increased to 100 mL / hr, per doctor's orders. Starting with the amount of IV fluid remaining at 1530, calculate the new infusion time and completion time of the IV.

   Infusion time_____

   Completion time_____

3. The doctor orders 1 L NS to infuse over 8 hours. The nurse starts the IV at 1600. At 2000, the IV rate is decreased to 100 mL / hr. Starting with the amount of IV fluid remaining at 2000, calculate the new infusion time and completion time of the IV.

Infusion time_____

Completion time_____

4. The doctor order 500 mL of NS to infuse at 100 mL / hr. The nurse starts the IV at 0530. At 0700, the IV rate is decreased to 75 mL / hr. Starting with the amount of IV fluid remaining at 0700, calculate the new infusion time and completion time of the IV.

Infusion time_____

Completion time_____

5. At 1600, 1 L D5W is started to infuse over 8 hours. At 1900, the IV infiltrates. The nurse restarts the IV at 2100 at the same IV rate. Starting with the amount of IV fluid remaining at 2100, calculate the new infusion time and completion time of the IV.

Infusion time_____

Completion time_____

Exercise: FOCUS ON SAFETY

Making Clinical Judgments in Working With Infusion and Completion Time

> - Read each situation, and then make a clinical judgment.
> - Provide a rationale for your decision or action.

SITUATION:

The nurse started 1 liter of D5/0.9% NS at 0700, to infuse at 125 mL / hr via gravity. The drop factor of the IV tubing is 15 gtt / mL. At 1200, the IV intake is 300 mL. In assessing the flow rate, the nurse counts 21 gtt / min. Which action(s) by the nurse are appropriate (select all that apply)?

a. Increase the flow rate to 31 gtt / min.

c. Report a completion time of 1736.

b. Increase the flow rate to 41 gtt / min for 4 hours.

d. Plan to give 1000 mL for the day shift.

e. Administer the IV fluid through an infusion pump.

Rationale / Discussion:

Labeling IV Bags
Label the following flowmeters to identify the IV fluid intake.

1. The doctor orders 1 L NS to infuse over 10 hours. The nurse starts the IV at 1100. Label the flowmeter with the hourly fluid intake.

```
Start
Time
 —    0
      __
 —100
      __
 —200
      __
 —300
      __
 —400
      __
 —500
      __
 —600
      __
 —700
      __
 —800
      __
 —900
      __
```

2. The nurse starts the IV at 0230, to infuse at 75 mL / hr. Label the flowmeter hourly.

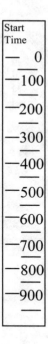

Start
Time

— 0

—100

—200

—300

—400

—500

—600

—700

—800

—900

3. The nurse starts the IV at 0100, at 50 mL / hr. Label the flowmeter q.2h.

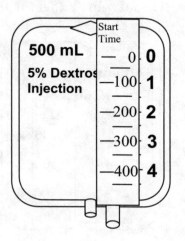

500 mL

5% Dextros
Injection

Start
Time

— 0   0

—100   1

—200   2

—300   3

—400   4

4. The nurse starts the IV at 1300, to infuse at
   150 mL / hr. Label the flowmeter hourly.

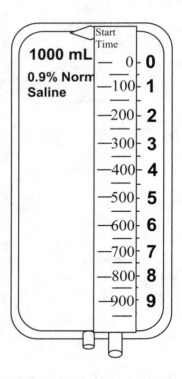

1000 mL

0.9% Norm Saline

Start Time

0	0
100	1
200	2
300	3
400	4
500	5
600	6
700	7
800	8
900	9

Shade in the
amount of IV
fluid in the
bag at 1700.

5. The nurse starts the IV at 2030 to infuse at
   125 mL / hr. Label the flowmeter hourly.

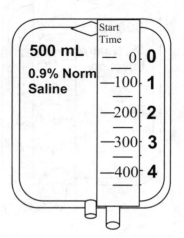

500 mL

0.9% Norm Saline

Start Time

0	0
100	1
200	2
300	3
400	4

Shade in the
amount of IV
fluid in the
bag at 2330.

Exercise: FOCUS ON SAFETY
Making Clinical Judgments in Working With Labeling IV Bags

- Read each situation, and then make a clinical judgment.
- Provide a rationale for your decision or action.

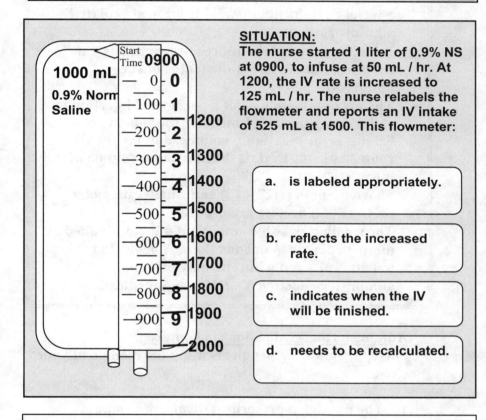

SITUATION:
The nurse started 1 liter of 0.9% NS at 0900, to infuse at 50 mL / hr. At 1200, the IV rate is increased to 125 mL / hr. The nurse relabels the flowmeter and reports an IV intake of 525 mL at 1500. This flowmeter:

a. is labeled appropriately.

b. reflects the increased rate.

c. indicates when the IV will be finished.

d. needs to be recalculated.

Rationale / Discussion:

Module: PEDIATRIC CALCULATIONS

ADMINISTERING MEDICATIONS TO CHILDREN

KEY POINTS:
- The oral route is preferred for children. Children over 5 years can take chewable forms of medication. Special equipment is available for oral pediatric administration.
- Parenteral doses for children are generally not rounded, but are left at the tenths or the hundredths place.
- The maximum volume of a parenteral injection in children is generally 1 mL. For the subcut route, 0.5 mL is the maximum volume, and for the ID route, 0.01 – 0. 1 mL is the maximum volume of the injection.
- Shorter length (1/2" – 1") and smaller diameter (25G – 30G) needles are used.
- The smallest possible amount of diluent is added to dilute pediatric IV medications. A pedidrip tubing (60 gtt / mL) and a burette may be used to administer pediatric IV fluids and medications.

Administering Medications to Children
Solve the following problems using the method of your choice.

1. The physician prescribed divalproex sodium 0.25 gram daily p.o. Divalproex sodium is available from the pharmacy in 125 mg delayed-release tablets. How many tablets will the nurse give?

_____

2. The child is to receive cefaclor 350 mg p.o. q.12h. The pharmacy sends strawberry-flavored cefaclor oral suspension in 125 mg / 5mL strength. How many mL will the child receive per dose?

_____

3. The doctor orders Diflucan® 60 mg b.i.d. The nurse finds the following in the medication drawer. How many mL will the nurse give?

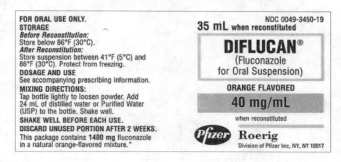

FOR ORAL USE ONLY.
STORAGE
Before Reconstitution:
Store below 86°F (30°C).
After Reconstitution:
Store suspension between 41°F (5°C) and 86°F (30°C). Protect from freezing.
DOSAGE AND USE
See accompanying prescribing information.
MIXING DIRECTIONS:
Tap bottle lightly to loosen powder. Add 24 mL of distilled water or Purified Water (USP) to the bottle. Shake well.
SHAKE WELL BEFORE EACH USE.
DISCARD UNUSED PORTION AFTER 2 WEEKS.
This package contains 1400 mg fluconazole in a natural orange-flavored mixture.*

NDC 0049-3450-19
35 mL when reconstituted

DIFLUCAN®
(Fluconazole
for Oral Suspension)

ORANGE FLAVORED
40 mg/mL
when reconstituted

Pfizer Roerig
Division of Pfizer Inc, NY, NY 10017

_____

4. The order is for 60 mg of Cleocin® p.o. q.i.d. for a 6-year-old child. The following medication is available. How many mL will the nurse give?

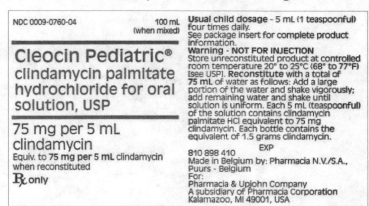

NDC 0009-0760-04
100 mL
(when mixed)

Cleocin Pediatric®
clindamycin palmitate hydrochloride for oral solution, USP

75 mg per 5 mL
clindamycin
Equiv. to **75 mg per 5 mL** clindamycin when reconstituted
℞ only

Usual child dosage - 5 mL (1 teaspoonful) four times daily.
See package insert for complete product information.
Warning - NOT FOR INJECTION
Store unreconstituted product at controlled room temperature 20° to 25°C (68° to 77°F) [see USP]. Reconstitute with a total of 75 mL of water as follows: Add a large portion of the water and shake vigorously; add remaining water and shake until solution is uniform. Each 5 mL (teaspoonful) of the solution contains clindamycin palmitate HCl equivalent to 75 mg clindamycin. Each bottle contains the equivalent of 1.5 grams clindamycin.
EXP
810 898 410
Made in Belgium by: Pharmacia N.V./S.A., Puurs - Belgium
For:
Pharmacia & Upjohn Company
A subsidiary of Pharmacia Corporation
Kalamazoo, MI 49001, USA

_____

5a. Prochlorperazine 2.5 mg p.o. b.i.d. is ordered. The pharmacy sends prochlorperazine syrup 5 mg / 5 mL. How many mL will the patient receive?

_____

b. Fill in the most appropriate measuring device for this medication.

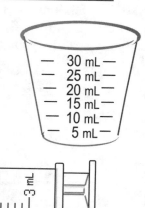

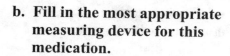

6a. Methylprednisolone 20 mg IV q.12h. is ordered. The pharmacy sends the following medication. How many mL will the nurse administer per dose?

| Solu-Medrol |
| Methylprednisolone USP |
| **125 mg / mL** |
| For IM or IV use |
| Single dose vial |

_____

b. Fill in the syringe.

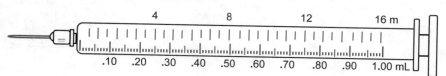

7. The physician orders IV tobramycin 12 mg q.12h. The pharmacy sends the following vial of tobramycin. How many mL will the nurse give?

> **Tobramycin sulfate injection**
>
> 20 mg per 2 mL
>
> For IM or IV use

_____

8a. The patient has a primary IV of D5/0.225% NS infusing by gravity flow at 75 mL / hr. The IV tubing is a pedidrip tubing. The physician orders ampicillin 250 mg in 50 mL D5W IV q.6h. The IVPB is to infuse over ½ hour. What is the flow rate of the IVPB?

_____

b. At what time will the IVPB be completed if the nurse starts the IVPB at 1400?

_____

9. The patient is to receive ampicillin 100 mg. After mixing the ampicillin, the nurse adds it to the volume control chamber and fills up the chamber with D5W to the 50 mL mark. The IV medication is to infuse over 60 minutes. How many mL / hr will the nurse set on the IV pump?

_____

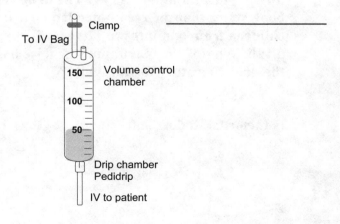

DETERMINING SAFE DOSE

KEY POINTS:

- In order to determine whether an ordered dose is safe for an individual child, the nurse needs the following information: the medication order, the child's weight (usually in kg) or body surface area (BSA), and the recommended dose from the drug reference book.
- Recommended drug dosages can be stated as individual doses (for example, mg / kg or mcg / m^2), total daily doses, or as dosage ranges. The nurse needs to read the drug reference book carefully to interpret the drug information correctly.
- After calculating the recommended dose based on a child's weight or BSA, it is compared with the ordered dose. An ordered dose is considered safe when it is equal to or smaller than the dose recommended in the drug reference book.

Dosage Based on Body Weight
Solve the following problems using the method of your choice.

1a. The physician orders cefdinir 200 mg p.o. q.12h., for a child who weighs 30 kg. The drug reference book states that the recommended dose for children from 6 months to 12 years is 7 mg / kg q.12h. What is the maximum safe dose based on the drug literature for this child?

_____

b. Is the ordered dose safe?

_____

2a. The physician orders a digitalizing dose of IV digoxin 0.25 mg p.o. q.12h., for a 12-month-old child who weighs 8 kg. The drug reference book states that the recommended digitalizing dose for children from 1 – 24 months is 30 – 50 mcg / kg. What is the maximum safe dose based on the drug literature for this child?

_____

  b. Is the ordered dose safe?

_____

3a. The physician orders furosemide oral solution 40 mg p.o. daily, for a child who weighs 66 lb. The drug reference book states that the recommended dose of p.o. furosemide for children is 1 – 2 mg / kg as a single dose initially, up to 5 – 6 mg / kg / day. What is the maximum safe dose based on the drug literature for this child?

_____

  b. Is the ordered dose safe?

_____

4a. A child who weighs 77 lb is started on oral morphine solution 20 mg p.o. q.3h. The recommended dose of oral morphine for children <50 kg is 0.3 mg / kg q.3 – 4h. initially. What is the maximum safe dose based on the drug literature for this child?

_____

  b. Is the ordered dose safe?

_____

5a. The order is for phenytoin sodium 125 mg IV q.8h., for a 15-year-old patient with frequent seizures. The patient weighs 55 kg. The drug reference book states that the recommended pediatric maintenance dose of phenytoin sodium is 4 – 8 mg / kg / 24 hr in divided doses every 8 – 12 hours. What is the maximum safe dose based on the drug literature for this child?

_____

b. Is the ordered dose safe?

_____

Dosage Based on Body Surface Area
Solve the following problems using the method of your choice.

1a. A child who has a BSA of 0.8 m^2 is given leucovorin calcium 5 mg q.6h. The drug reference book states that the recommended dose for children is 7 mg / m^2 q.6h. What is the maximum safe dose based on the drug literature for this child?

_____

b. Is the ordered dose safe?

_____

2a. An order is written for zidovudine 0.25 g p.o. q.6h., for a child who has a BSA of 1.1 m^2. The drug reference book states that the recommended dose for children from 3 months to 12 years is 90 – 180 mg / m^2 q.6h. What is the maximum safe dose based on the drug literature for this child?

_____

b. Is the ordered dose safe?

_____

3a. The physician prescribes vinblastine 10 mg IV q.week, for a child who weighs 75 lb and has a body surface area of 1.15 m^2. The drug reference book states that the recommended dose of vinblastine for children is 2.5 mg / m^2 as a single dose initially, up to 7.5 mg / m^2/ q.1 – 2 weeks up to 12 weeks. What is the maximum safe dose based on the drug literature for this child?

_____

b. Is the ordered dose safe?

_____

4a. The order is for 0.2 mg q.AM of a drug for a child with a BSA of 0.4 m^2. The recommended dose of the drug is 0.55 mg / m^2 daily. What is the maximum safe dose based on the drug literature for this child?

_____

b. Is the ordered dose safe?

_____

5a. An 11-year-old child with leukemia and an acute varicella zoster infection is started on acyclovir 500 mg IV q.8h. The child's BSA is 1.18 m^2. The recommended dose of acyclovir for immunosuppressed children <12 years old with varicella zoster is 500 mg / m^2 q.8h. for 7 days. What is the maximum safe dose based on the drug literature for this child?

_____

b. Is the ordered dose safe?

_____

Exercise: FOCUS ON SAFETY

Making Clinical Judgments in Working With Determining Safe Dose

- Read each situation, and then make a clinical judgment.
- Provide a rationale for your decision or action.

Date	Physician's Orders
2/15	Lamotrigine 35 mg p.o. B.I.D.

Patient M
ID *******

SITUATION:
The physician is starting lamotrigine drug therapy on a child who weighs 27 kg.

The drug reference book states that the recommended initial pediatric dose of lamotrigine is 0.6 mg / kg / day in 2 divided doses for the first two weeks.

Which action by the nurse is most appropriate?

a. administer the medication as ordered.

c. ask the pharmacist if the ordered dose is correct.

b. question the ordered dose.

d. ask the parent what dose the child has been taking.

Rationale / Discussion:

NASOGASTRIC FLUID REPLACEMENT

KEY POINTS:

- To calculate fluid replacement for a child with a large volume of NG drainage, the nurse needs the following information: the rate of the primary IV, the maximum hourly IV rate, the amount of NG drainage, and the time interval for measuring and replacing the output.
- NG fluid replacement problems usually involve solving for the infusion and completion time of the replacement IV fluid.

Working With Nasogastric Fluid Replacement Problems
Solve the following problems using the method of your choice.

1a. An adolescent patient with a NG tube set to low continuous suction has an order for 1 L D5/0.225% NS @ 100 mL / hr. The NG drainage is to be measured q.8h. and replaced with a second IV of D5W with 10 mEq KCl per 500 mL. The patient is to receive no more than 150 mL / hr IV. What is the rate of the primary IV?

_____

b. What is the maximum hourly IV rate?

_____

c. The patient's NG tube drains 380 mL. What is the infusion time of the replacement IV?

_____

d. What is the completion time of the replacement IV if replacement is started at 1500?

_____

2a. The order is for 500 mL D5/0.225% NS @ 63 mL / hr. The NG drainage is to be measured and replaced with the primary IV solution q.4h. Maximum hourly IV rate is not to exceed 85 mL / hr. What is the rate of the primary IV?

_____

b. The nurse can increase the IV by how many additional mL / hr during the replacement of the NG drainage?

_____

c. The child's NG tube drains 66 mL. What is the infusion time of the replacement IV fluid?

_____

d. The fluid replacement is started at 12 noon. What is the completion time?

_____

3a. The physician writes the following orders:
1. IV 500 mL 0.33% NS @ 75 mL / hr.
2. Replace NG drainage mL for mL q.4h. with 2nd IV of 0.45% NS with 10 mEq KCl per 500 mL.
3. Maximum hourly IV rate 100 mL / hr.
The NG output at 0400 is 100 mL. What is the infusion time of the replacement IV?

_____

b. What is the completion time if the replacement IV is started at 0430?

_____

4a. The physician writes the following orders:
   1. IV 500 mL D5/0.225% NS q.10h.
   2. Replace NG drainage mL for mL with the maintenance IV fluid q.4h.
   3. Maximum hourly IV rate 80 mL / hr.
   The NG output at 2200 is 135 mL. What is the infusion time of the replacement IV fluid?

   _____

   b. What is the completion time if the replacement IV is started at 2245?

   _____

5a. The physician writes the following orders:
   1. IV 250 mL D5/ 0.9% NS at 25 mL / hr.
   2. Replace NG drainage mL for mL q.4h.
   3. Maximum hourly IV rate 50 mL / hr.
   The NG output at 1500 is 65 mL. What is the infusion time of the replacement IV fluid?

   _____

   b. What is the completion time if the replacement IV is started at 1600?

   _____

6a. The physician writes the following orders:
   1. IV 250 mL D5W at 40 mL / hr.
   2. Replace NG drainage mL for mL with the maintenance IV fluid q.8h.
   3. Maximum hourly IV rate 75 mL / hr.
   The NG output at 0600 is 115 mL. What is the infusion time of the replacement IV fluid?

   _____

   b. What is the completion time if the replacement IV is started at 0700?

   _____

Module: TITRATION OF IV MEDICATIONS

TITRATION OF IV MEDICATIONS

KEY POINTS:

- With titration problems, the nurse usually needs to calculate the number of mL / hr to set on the IV pump. Occasionally, the nurse must calculate the amount of medication infusing per hour.
- Information needed to solve titration problems includes the total drug, the total volume of IV fluid, and the amount of drug ordered to infuse hourly.
- Titration orders can be written as a dosage range or as a single dose of medication.

Titration in Common Clinical Practice
Solve the following titration problems.

1. Heparin 25,000 units in 250 mL D5W is sent up from the pharmacy. The order is to administer heparin at 1000 units / hr. How many mL / hr will the nurse set on the IV pump?

   _____

2. The pharmacy sends an IV of 125 mg diltiazem HCl in 500 mL D5W. The physician has ordered diltiazem HCl 5 mg / hr. Calculate the mL / hr.

   _____

3. One gram of aminophylline is added to 500 mL NS. The order is to infuse the IV over 10 hours. Calculate the mg / hr that the patient will receive.

   _____

4. The doctor writes an order for heparin 1400 units / hr. The pharmacy sends an IV of 500 mL D5W with 20,000 units of heparin. What rate will the nurse set on the IV pump?

   _____

5. The physician orders IV morphine sulfate
   2 – 5 mg / hr for pain management. The pharmacy
   sends an IV of 250 mg of morphine sulfate in 500
   mL D5W. What rate will the nurse set on the IV
   pump to administer 3 mg / hr?

   _____

6a. A patient with severe asthma who weighs 55 kg is
    started on an IV theophylline drip in the
    emergency room. An IV of 250 mg theophylline
    ethylenediamine in 500 mL NS is started at 1300.
    The order is to start the IV infusion
    at 0.5 mg / kg / hr. The dose to be increased as
    needed by 0.1 mg / kg / hr q.30 min, up to a
    maximum of 0.7 mg / kg / hr. Calculate the
    mL / hr that the nurse will set on the infusion
    pump at 1300.

    _____

 b. If the theophylline drip is increased as ordered at
    1330, what rate will be set on the IV pump?

    _____

Complex Titration Problems in Critical Care
Solve the following titration problems.

1. Ordered: IV dobutamine 100 mcg / min
   Available: dobutamine 250 mg in 250 mL D5W
   The nurse is told in the morning report that the
   patient is receiving 5 mL / hr via IV pump.

   a. Calculate the mg / hr.

      _____

   b. Calculate the mL / hr.

      _____

   c. Is the set rate correct?

      _____

Copyright © 2007, F. A. Davis Company

2. Ordered: 1 mg lidocaine / min IV
   Available: 2 g lidocaine in 500 mL D5W

   a. Calculate the mg / hr.

   _____

   b. Calculate the mL / hr.

   _____

   c. If the lidocaine is increased to 2 mg / min,
       calculate the mL / hr.

   _____

3. Ordered: IV lidocaine 4 mg / min
   Available: 1 g lidocaine in 500 mL D5W

   a. Calculate the mL / hr.

   _____

   b. If the rate is reduced to 2 mg / min, calculate the
      mL / hr.

   _____

4. The pharmacy sends an IV of magnesium sulfate
   22 gram in 500 mL D5W. The order is for
   50 mg / min. Calculate the mL / hr.

   _____

5. A patient with ventricular ectopic beats has stat
   orders for a lidocaine infusion at a rate of
   30 mL / hr. The IV contains 1 g lidocaine in 500
   mL D5W. Calculate the mg / hr that the patient
   will receive.

   _____

6. Pronestyl® 1 gram in 250 mL NS is ordered for a
   patient with frequent PVCs, to run at 1 mL / min.
   Calculate the mg / min that the patient is receiving.

   _____

7. The order is for IV dopamine HCl 400 mg in 500 mL NS. The patient is to receive 750 mcg / min. What rate will the nurse set on the IV pump?

   _____

8. Ordered: Nitroglycerine 10 mcg / min IV
   Available: Nitroglycerine 50 mg in 250 mL NS
   What rate will the nurse set on the IV pump?

   _____

9. The order is for IV dopamine HCl 400 mg / 500 mL NS. The patient is to receive 500 – 750 mcg / min. What rate will the nurse set on the IV pump to administer the lowest dosage of dopamine HCl?

   _____

10. The order is for IV NTG 5 – 100 mcg / min to relieve chest pain. NTG 50 mg in 250 mL NS is available. What rate will the nurse set on the IV pump to deliver the highest dosage?

    _____

11. The physician orders dopamine 20 mcg / kg / min for a patient who weighs 80 kg. The pharmacy sends an IV of 400 mg of dopamine in 500 mL D5W. What rate will the nurse set on the IV pump?

    _____

12. The physician orders milrinone lactate 0.5 – 0.75 mcg / kg / min IV for a patient with CHF who weighs 121 lb. The pharmacy sends an IV of 20 mg of milrinone lactate in 150 mL D5W. What rate will the nurse set on the IV pump to administer the lowest dosage?

    _____

13. The physician orders propranolol 1 mg / hr. The pharmacy sends an IV of 15 mg propranolol in 500 mL NS. Calculate the mL / hr.

_____

14a. The patient has a dopamine drip running at 45 mL / hr. The order is for 400 mg dopamine HCl in 500 mL D5W to run at 5 – 15 mcg / kg / min. The dopamine is started at 8 mcg / kg / min. The patient weighs 165 pounds. Is the correct rate set on the IV pump?

_____

b. If the rate is increased to 9 mcg / kg / min, what rate should be set on the IV pump?

_____

Exercise: FOCUS ON SAFETY

Making Clinical Judgments in Working With Titration Medication

- Read each situation, and then make a clinical judgment.
- Provide a rationale for your decision or action.

Date	Physician's Orders
7/10	Start D5W 500 mL with 20,000 units heparin. Heparin to infuse at 1100 units every hour. Patient C ID *******

SITUATION:
To carry out this order safely, the nurse would (select all that apply):

a. set the infusion rate at _____ mL / hr.

b. set the infusion rate at _____ gtt / min.

c. use a minidrop IV tubing for gravity flow infusion.

d. set up the IV using an infusion pump.

e. discontinue the IV once the 500 mL have infused.

Rationale / Discussion:

ANSWERS

Module: BASIC MATH REVIEW

Working With Addition of Fractions (pp. 1 – 2)

1.	3/5	6.	15 5/24
2.	11/21	7.	14 4/45
3.	1 1/15	8.	15 1/10
4.	5 1/4	9.	17 5/8
5.	5 9/20	10.	21 3/4

Working With Subtraction of Fractions (p. 2)

1.	1/2	6.	2 1/2
2.	3/10	7.	4 21/40
3.	5/24	8.	10 11/24
4.	2 7/8	9.	10 19/42
5.	7 3/10	10.	7 1/10

Working With Multiplication of Fractions (p. 3)

1.	3/10	6.	14 16/21
2.	5/9	7.	3 3/16
3.	1/2	8.	11 11/35
4.	15/16	9.	22 11/24
5.	19 4/5	10.	3 13/54

Working With Division of Fractions (pp. 3 – 4)

1.	1 2/5	6.	12/29
2.	1/50	7.	11/20
3.	1 1/4	8.	1 13/15
4.	9 3/7	9.	33
5.	14/15	10.	22/35

Working With Addition of Decimals (pp. 4 – 5)

1.	6074.6132		7.	21.62
2.	142.205		8.	59.52
3.	1.988		9.	65.71
4.	1961.1713		10.	28.99
5.	56.97		11.	35.99
6.	70.8		12.	28.12

Working With Subtraction of Decimals (pp. 5 – 6)

1.	321.0155		7.	423.697
2.	0.051		8.	66.8
3.	9012.333		9.	8703.8
4.	7049.263		10.	853.1
5.	7.977		11.	553.9
6.	601.05		12.	939.2

Working With Multiplication of Decimals (p. 6)

1.	75.28		7.	3.6888
2.	1.6168		8.	7.344
3.	336.742		9.	320.1
4.	78.0861		10.	0.2475
5.	0.102		11.	67.6208
6.	30.1515		12.	50.47

Working With Division of Decimals (pp. 6 – 7)

1.	45		7.	48.1
2.	112		8.	83.4
3.	7.08		9.	46.7
4.	20.5		10.	0.0565
5.	0.05		11.	49.456
6.	401.2		12.	1.084

Working With Roman Numerals (p. 8)

1.	VIISS		5.	CI
2.	XXXV		6.	XVSS
3.	XLI		7.	XCIX
4.	LXV		8.	MMXI

Working With Roman Numerals (p. 9)

1. 30
2. 14
3. 49
4. 1 1/2
5. 150
6. 95
7. 75
8. 2010

Module: METHODS OF CALCULATION

Working With Methods of Calculation (pp. 10 – 15)

1. 2 tablets
2. 1 ½ tablets
3. 2 pills
4. 0.5 tablet
5. 3 caplets
6. 3.5 mL
7. 6 mL
8. 0.5 mL
9. 3 mL
10. 16 mL
11. 10 days
12. 10 days
13. 2.25 mL
14. 3.5 mL
15. 30 mL
16. 0.6 mL
17. 15 days
18. 20 mL
19a. 0.4 mL
  b. 5 doses
20a. 0.8 mL
  b. 5 doses
  c. 0.65 mL
  d. 6 doses

Module: SYSTEMS OF MEASUREMENT

Working With the Metric System (pp. 16 – 18)

1. 3500 mL
2. 700 mL
3. 1 g
4. 0.1 mg
5. 10,000 mcg
6. 2000 mcg
7. 0.0356 g
8. 0.00745 L
9. 0.007 dm
10. 10,000 M
11. 1000 mm
12. 1650 g
13. 1.5 L
14. 2500 mg
15. 0.75 g
16. 500 mg
17. 0.075 mg
18. 450 mcg
19. 1200 g
20. 40 mm
21. 1.4 mL
22. 10 mL
23. 0.5 mL
24. 20 mL
25. 1.5 tablets
26. 0.25 mL

Working With the Household System (pp. 19 – 20)

1. 6 tsp
2. 2 T
3. 3 tsp
4. 16 oz
5. 8 oz
6. 4.4 lb
7. 1 T

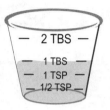

8. 10 mL

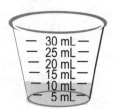

9. 24 oz
10. 8 oz

Working With Conversions Between Systems (pp. 21 – 22)

1. 15 mL
2. 0.001 mg
3. 1 oz
4. 30 mcg
5. 1750 mg
6. 500 mg
7. 1.5 oz
8. 5 tsp
9. 0.085 g
10. 2 mL
11. 4 t
12. 9 t
13. 480 mL
14. 2.54 cm
15. 10 mm
16. 165 lb
17. 90 kg
18. 0.3 L
19. 2 tablets
20. 360 mL
21. 184.8 lb
22. 2 tablets
23. 3 tsp
24. 0.3 mL
25. 0.75 mL

Module: INTAKE AND OUTPUT

Working With Intake and Output (pp. 23 – 27)

1.   I 960 mL
       O 440 mL

2.   I 270 mL
       O 280 mL

3.   O 1410 mL

4.   I 300 mL
       O 270 mL

5.   I 2020 mL
       O 595 mL

6.   I 1000 mL

7.   I 1224 mL
       O 425 mL

8.   I 1330 mL
       O 605 mL

9.   I 970 mL
       O 480 mL

10. I 675 mL

11. I 1660 mL
        O 800 mL

12. I 750 mL
        O 1125 mL

13. I 375 mL

Exercise: FOCUS ON SAFETY
Making Clinical Judgments in Working With Intake and Output (p. 28)

c. question the documented amount of the IVPBs.
CORRECT: *The documented parenteral intake identifies the primary IV intake (600 mL) for the day shift and an IVPB intake of 100 mL. Each IVPB contained 100 mL. The day nurse reported that two IVPBs were given.*

INCORRECT:
a. question the recorded 100 mL urine output.
The situation does not indicate any reason to question the 100 mL output.
b. recalculate the primary IV intake.
The primary IV has infused appropriately for the shift.
d. plan to administer an IVPB of KCl.
The nurse should clarify if the IVPB was given before planning the administration of another dose.

Working With Nasogastric Tube Feeding Problems (pp. 29 – 31)

1. 80 mL
2. 466 mL
3. 119 mL
4. 750 mL
5. 237 mL
6. 711 mL
7. 200 mL
8. 79 mL
9. 500 mL
10. 120 mL

Exercise: FOCUS ON SAFETY
Making Clinical Judgments in Working With Nasogastric Tube Feeding (p. 32)

b. The amount of water added to the formula.

CORRECT: *The ordered formula strength is 2/3. The nurse starts with 200 mL of formula. To make a 2/3-strength formula, the nurse needs to add 100 mL of water, not 80 mL.*

INCORRECT:
a. The documented N/G tube intake should be 400 mL.
The documented N/G tube intake is correct.
c. The IV intake is incorrect for the ordered rate.
The documented IV intake is correct.
d. The formula strength should be questioned.
The formula strength is ordered by the physician.

Module: READING MEDICATION LABELS

Working With Reading Medication Labels (pp. 33 –38)

1. a. Precose
   b. acarbose
   c. 100 mg / tablet
   d. tablet
   e. oral

Copyright © 2007, F. A. Davis Company

2.   a. fentanyl citrate
      b. 100 mcg / 2 mL
        50 mcg / mL
        0.05 mg / mL
      c. liquid for injection (milliliters)
      d. IV or IM
      e. Yes
      f. single-dose
      g. 1.5 mL

3.   a. Cipro
      b. ciprofloxacin
      c. dilute with 100 to 200 mL of suitable diluent

4.   a. morphine sulfate
      b. 5 mg / 10 mL
        0.5 mg / mL
      c. 10 mL
      d. IV, Epidural or Intrathecal
      e. Yes
      f. Yes
      g. 6 mL

5.   a. 7.5 mL

6.   a. midazolam hydrochloride
      b. 25 mg / 5 mL
        5 mg / mL
      c. IM or IV
      d. Yes
      e. No
      f. 2.5 mL

7.   a. Corvert
      b. 1 mg / 10 mL
        0.1 mg / mL
      c. IV use only
      d. store at controlled room temperature

8. a. 1.25 mg / mL
    b. IV
    c. No
    d. 0.5 mL

9. a. 40 mcg / mL

10. a. NPH Iletin II
    b. Purified Pork

11. a. Humalog
    b. 6 units

12. a. Novolin 70/30
    b. 22 units

13. a. Humulin 50/50
    b. 17 units

Exercise: FOCUS ON SAFETY
Making Clinical Judgments in Working With
Reading Medication Labels (p. 39)

d. not administer this drug.

CORRECT: *The order is for morphine, not hydromorphone. Although both drugs are opioid analgesics, they are different drugs. The nurse needs to ensure that the available drug corresponds to what is ordered.*

INCORRECT:
a. give 1.5 mL of the prefilled syringe.
Before calculating how much medication to give, the nurse should ensure that correct drug is being prepared. The order is for morphine, not hydromorphone.
b. call the pharmacist to double check the order.
The nurse should first check the original order found in the Physician's Order sheet.
c. research the appropriate route of administration.
Although this is important, the nurse should first ensure that the available drug corresponds to what is ordered.

Module: ORAL MEDICATIONS

Working With Oral Medications (pp. 40 – 45)

1.	2 tablets	13.	5 days
2.	1/2 tablet	14.	1/2 tablet
3.	2 tablets	15.	1 tablet
4.	2 tablets	16.	10 mL
5.	2 tablets	17.	12.5 mL
6.	960 mg	18.	2 tab (6.25mg)
7.	8 mL	19.	720 mg
8.	2 tsp	20.	1 tablespoon
9.	20 mL	21.	3 tablets
10.	1 tablet	22.	30 mL
11.	10 mL	23.	1 tsp
12.	2 tablets	24.	lanoxin 0.5 tablet
			Captopril 1 tablet
			furosemide 2 tabs

Exercise: FOCUS ON SAFETY
Making Clinical Judgments in Working With Oral Medications (p. 46)

b. Call the pharmacist regarding the propranolol.
CORRECT: *The nurse should call the pharmacist to clarify the propranolol 60 mg ER found in the patient's medication drawer.*
d. Give the hydralazine and the K-Dur at 0900.
CORRECT: *The nurse can administer the 0900 hydralazine and the K-Dur to the patient. The nurse should not administer the propranolol until it is clarified.*

INCORRECT:
a. Give all the 0900 medications.
The nurse should question the propranolol 60 mg ER prior to administering the drug.
c. Call the pharmacist regarding the K-Dur.
The K-Dur may be given as ordered.
e. Give the hydralazine and propranolol at 0900.
The nurse should hold and question the administration of the propranolol 60 mg ER.

Module: SYRINGES AND NEEDLES

Working With Syringes (pp. 47 – 50)

1. **0.3 mL**

2. **0.66 mL**

3. **0.09 mL**

4. **7.5 minims**

5. **15 minims**

6. **1.2 mL**

7. **2.7 mL**

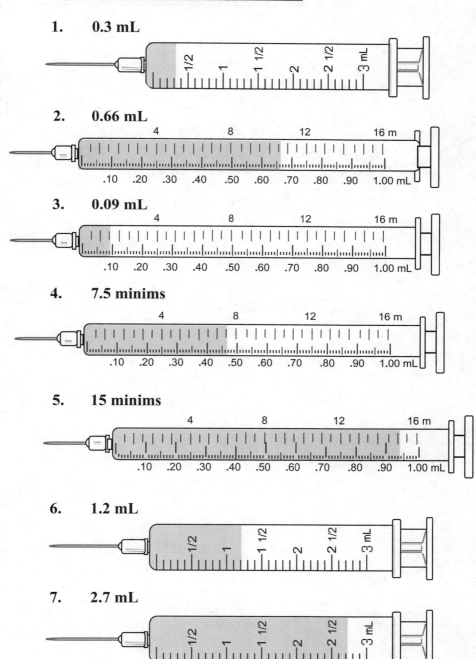

8. **0.37 mL**

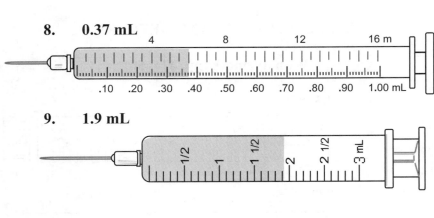

9. **1.9 mL**

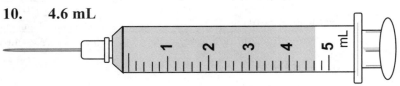

10. **4.6 mL**

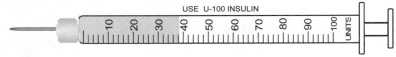

11. **38 units**

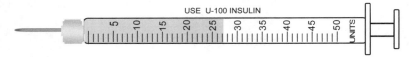

12. **27 units**

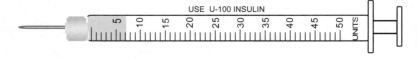

13. **7 units**

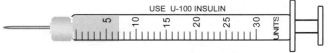

14. **7 units**

15.   16 units

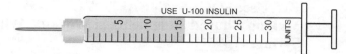

16.   56 units

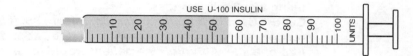

17.   72 units

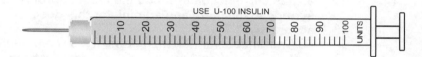

18.   3.8 mL

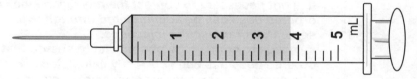

19.   0.5 mL

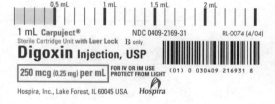

20.   1.5 mL

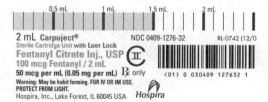

Exercise: FOCUS ON SAFETY
Making Clinical Judgments in Working With
Syringes (p. 51)

d. should divide the medication into two injections using two 3 mL syringes.
CORRECT: *For intramuscular (IM) injections, it is recommended that no more than 3 mL be administered into one site. Although the patient would receive two injections, this is the safest action.*

INCORRECT:
a. has correctly determined the most appropriate syringe to measure and administer this dose accurately.
For intramuscular (IM) injections, it is recommended that no more than 3 mL be administered into one site.
b. needs to contact the physician and request a higher dosage strength of the medication.
It is not necessary to contact the physician since the ordered dose can be administered through two separate intramuscular injections.
c. needs to contact the pharmacist to ensure that the ordered dose has been correctly calculated.
The nurse can ask another professional nurse to check the calculation.

Working With Needles (p. 52)

1.   28G ½" or 31G 5/16"
2.   21 – 23G 1 ½"
3.   26 – 27G 3/8"
4.   21 – 23G 2"
5.   25G 5/8"
6.   18 – 19G 1"

Working With Needles (pp. 53 – 55)

1. **Meperidine 75 mg (1 mL) IM**

b.

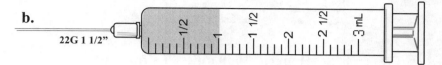

22G 1 1/2"

2. **Filgrastim 300 mcg (1 mL) subcut**

b.

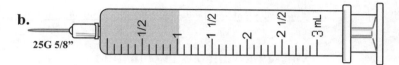

25G 5/8"

3. **Heparin 5,000 units (0.67 mL) subcut**

a.

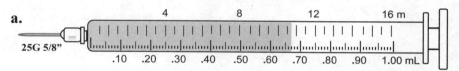

25G 5/8"

4. **Hepatitis A vaccine 1 mL IM**

b.

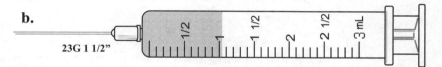

23G 1 1/2"

5. **Ketorolac 60 mg (2 mL) IM**

b.

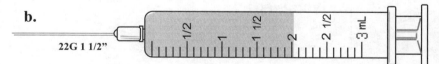

22G 1 1/2"

6. **Regular insulin 17 units subcut**

a.

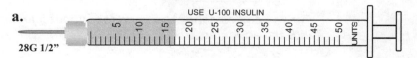

28G 1/2"

7. Regular insulin 6 units and NPH insulin 13 units subcut

a.

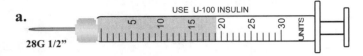

28G 1/2"

8. Heparin 1000 units (0.1 mL) subcut

a.

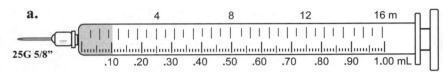

25G 5/8"

9. Morphine sulfate 1 mg (16 minims) subcut

b.

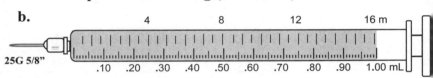

25G 5/8"

Exercise: FOCUS ON SAFETY
Making Clinical Judgments in Working With Needles
(p. 56)

d.

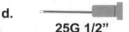

25G 1/2"

CORRECT: *Medications ordered via the subcut route
are meant to be injected into the adipose tissue.
A 25G ½" needle will appropriately administer the
ordered medication into the correct site.*

INCORRECT:

a.   18G 1"

b.

20G 1 ½"

c.

22G 1"

*These needles cannot be used for subcut injections
into the abdomen.*

Module: PARENTERAL MEDICATIONS

Working With Parenteral Medications (pp. 57 – 64)

1. 0.2 mL
2. 1.5 mL
3. 0.25 mL
4. 2 mL

Fill in the syringe.

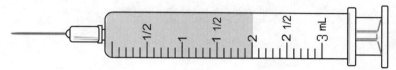

5. morphine sulfate   = 0.6 mL
   glycopyrrolate   = 0.4 mL

   Total amount   = 1 mL
   Fill in the syringe with the total amount.

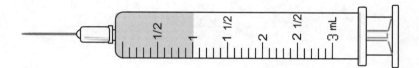

6. 0.1 mL
   Fill in the syringe.

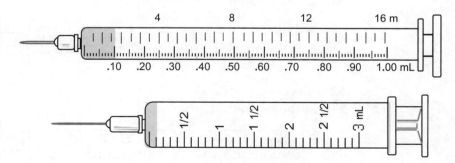

7. 0.4 mL

8. **16 minims**

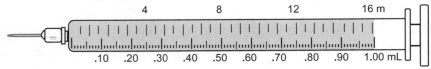

9. **0.6 mL**
Fill in the ordered dose in each syringe.

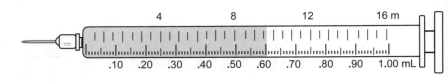

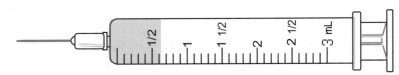

10. **0.25 mL**
Fill in the syringe.

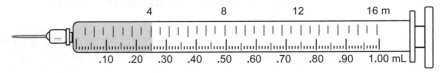

11. **2.5 mL**

12. **23 units**
Fill in the syringe.

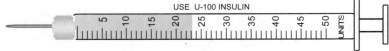

13. **52 units**
Fill in the syringe.

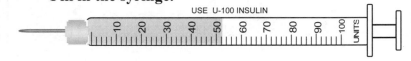

14. 21 units
Fill in the syringe.

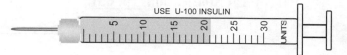

15. 19 units
Fill in the syringe.

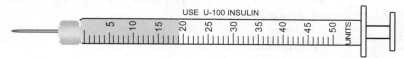

16. 2 units
Fill in the syringe.

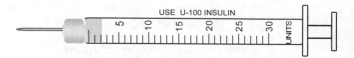

17. 29 units
Fill in the syringe.

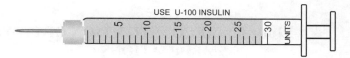

18. 0.9 mL

19. 1.2 mL

20. 0.8 mL

21. 0.5 mL

22. 1 mL

23. 0.5 mL

d. 1.63 mL

CORRECT: *The dosage strength of levothyroxine is 40 mcg / mL. The ordered dose is 0.065 mg, which is equivalent to 65 mcg.*

INCORRECT:
a. 0.33 mL
Use the dosage strength of 40 mcg / mL as listed under the Usual Dosage information.
b. 1.38 mL
Use the dosage strength of 40 mcg / mL as listed under the Usual Dosage information.
c. 1.5 mL
Use the dosage strength of 40 mcg / mL as listed under the Usual Dosage information.

Module: RECONSTITUTION OF POWDERED MEDICATIONS

Working With Single-Strength Reconstitution (pp. 66 – 70)

1.a. 2.5 mL
  b. sterile water for injection
  c. 330 mg / mL
  d. 0.76 mL

2.a. 4.6 mL
  b. bacteriostatic water for injection
  c. 200,000 units / mL
  d. 1.5 mL

3. date and time of reconstitution; nurse's initials

4.a. 2 mL
  b. sterile water for injection
  c. 125 mg / mL
  d. 1.6 mL

5.a. 1 g / 2.6 mL
  b. 1.3 mL

6.a. 2 mL
  b. sterile water for injection
  c. 225 mg / 1 mL
  d. 2 mL

7.a. 87 mL
  b. 250 mg / 5 mL
  c. 10 mL
  d. date and time of reconstitution; nurse's initials

8.   1.7 mL

Exercise: FOCUS ON SAFETY
Making Clinical Judgments in Working With Single-Strength Reconstitution (p. 71)

c.   Question the date of reconstitution.

CORRECT: *Although the nurse's initials and time of reconstitution are written, the date of reconstitution is not written on the Augmentin label. The nurse needs to clarify this prior to administering the drug to the patient.*

INCORRECT:
a.   Convert the tsp to mL.
The nurse may want to do this prior to administration, however, it is more important to first clarify the date of reconstitution.
b.   Administer the measured dose.
The nurse must first clarify the date of reconstitution.
d.   Use a 3 mL syringe to measure the dose.
It is more important to first clarify the date of reconstitution.

Working With Multiple-Strength Reconstitution (pp. 72 – 76)

1.   the smallest volume of diluent

2.a.   100 mg / mL
   b.   7.5 mL
   c.   date and time of reconstitution; nurse's initials; circle selected volume of diluent and corresponding dosage strength

3.a.   100,000 units / mL
   b.   500,000 units / mL
   c.   9.6 mL of diluent – give 10 mL
       4.6 mL of diluent – give 5 mL
       1.6 mL of diluent – give 2 mL

4.a.   75 mL of diluent – 250,000 units / mL
       33 mL of diluent – 500,000 units / mL
       11.5 mL of diluent – 1,000,000 units / mL
   b.   75 mL of diluent – give 3 mL
       33 mL of diluent – give 1.5 mL
       11.5 mL of diluent – give 0.75 mL
   c.   7 days
   d.   date and time of reconstitution; nurse's initials; circle selected volume of diluent and corresponding dosage strength
5.a.   3.5 mL of diluent – 500 mg / mL
       7.2 mL of diluent – 250 mg / mL
   b.   3.5 mL of diluent – give 1.4 mL
       7.2 mL of diluent – give 2.8 mL
   c.   1 hour at room temperature; 6 hours under refrigeration
   d.   3.5 mL is preferable so that the volume of the IM injection is smaller.
   e.   date and time of reconstitution; nurse's initials; circle selected volume of diluent and the corresponding dosage strength

6.a.   After reading the label, the nurse can
        identify the (check all that apply):
        ☒ routes of administration
        ☒ storage information
        ☒ usual adult dosage

  b.   To administer the ordered dose (500 mg), the
        nurse:
        ☒ should read the accompanying
          literature.

Exercise: FOCUS ON SAFETY
Making Clinical Judgments in Working With
Multiple-Strength Reconstitution (p. 77)

b. Recalculate the dose drawn up.

CORRECT: *The circle around the dosage strength*
indicates that the drug has already been
reconstituted. The reconstituted drug yields 500,000
units / mL. The order is for 2,400,000 units. After
calculating, the nurse will draw up 4.8 mL.

INCORRECT:
a. Add the 5 mL to the IV bag.
The order is for 2,400,000 units. After calculating,
the answer is 4.8 mL. The nurse can accurately
measure this dose using a 5 mL syringe.
c. Add 9.6 mL of penicillin G potassium to the IV
    bag.
The nurse needs to use the reconstituted dosage
strength that is circled on the label.
d. Use 1,000,000 U / mL to calculate the desired
    dose.
The nurse needs to use the reconstituted dosage
strength that is circled on the label.

Module: IV CALCULATIONS

Working With Milliliters per Hour (pp. 78 – 79)

1.   83 mL / hr
2.   63 mL / hr

3. 125 mL / hr
4. 167 mL / hr
5. 100 mL / hr
6. 167 mL / hr
7. 50 mL / hr
8. 138 mL / hr
9. 100 mL / hr
10. 133 mL / hr

Working With Flow Rate (p. 80 – 81)

1. 125 gtt / min
2. 21 gtt / min
3. 21 gtt / min
4. 8 gtt / min
5. 11 gtt / min
6. 33 gtt / min
7. 31 gtt / min
8. 167 gtt /min
9. 26 gtt / min
10. 25 gtt / min

Exercise: FOCUS ON SAFETY
Making Clinical Judgments in Working With Milliliters per Hour and Flow Rate (p. 82)

a. continue to monitor the IV intake at 13 gtt / min.

CORRECT: *The IV is set at the appropriate rate to deliver 50 mL / hr.*

INCORRECT:
b. question the oral intake for the day shift.
   There is no indication for questioning the oral intake in this situation.
c. increase the flow rate to 31 gtt / min.
   The IV rate is accurate and should not be increased without an MD order.
d. change the IV tubing to a minidrop.
   The IV tubing does not need to be changed. The flow rate can be accurately set and monitored with the current tubing.

Working With IV Push Medications (pp. 83 – 85)

1. 4 – 5 minutes
2. 6 – 10 minutes
3. 1 – 2 minutes
4. 2 – 3 minutes
5. 2 minutes
6. 1 minute
7. 2 minutes or longer (3 minutes or 8 – 15 minutes)

Exercise: FOCUS ON SAFETY
Making Clinical Judgments in Working With Milliliters per Hour and Flow Rate (p. 86)

> b. administer 0.8 mL over 2 minutes.
>
> **CORRECT:**
> *The recommended rate of administration is 0.6 mg over 1 minute. The order is for 0.8 mg, which will require an additional minute for administration.*
>
> **INCORRECT:**
> a. give the ordered dose slowly into the vein.
> *For safe administration, the nurse needs to follow the recommended rate and routes of administration.*
> c. add the atropine dose to the primary IV fluid.
> *The order is for IVP. The atropine should not be added to the primary IV fluid.*
> d. Dilute with 10 mL normal saline.
> *The recommended solution for dilution is sterile water.*

Working With Infusion Time (pp. 87 – 88)

1. 8 hours
2. 8 hours 20 minutes
3. 13 hours 20 minutes
4. 6 hours 24 minutes
5. 30 minutes
6. 3 hours 20 minutes

Working With Completion Time (pp. 88 – 89)
1. 4:00 PM or 1600
2. 6:10 PM or 1810
3. 6:00 AM or 0600
4. 3:30 AM or 0330
5. 8:45 PM or 2045
6. 2:00 PM or 1400

Working With Infusion and Completion Time (pp. 89 – 90)
1. Infusion Time = 9 hours
   Completion Time = 8:00 PM or 2000
2. Infusion Time = 3 hours 30 minutes
   Completion Time = 7:00 PM or 1900
3. Infusion Time = 5 hours
   Completion Time = 1:00 AM or 0100
4. Infusion Time = 4 hours 40 minutes
   Completion Time = 11:40 AM or 1140
5. Infusion Time = 5 hours
   Completion Time = 2:00 AM or 0200

Exercise: FOCUS ON SAFETY
Making Clinical Judgments in Working With Infusion and Completion Time (p. 91)

a. Increase the flow rate to 31 gtt / min.
CORRECT: *The nurse should increase the correct flow rate to administer 125 mL / hr.*
c. Report a completion time of 1736.
CORRECT: *At 1200, there are 700 mL of fluid left in the primary IV. Following the physician's orders to administer 125 mL / hr, It will take 5 hr and 36 minutes for 700 mL to infuse into the patient.*

INCORRECT:
b. Increase the flow rate to 41 gtt / min for 4 hours.
The flow rate should not be adjusted to "catch up."
d. Plan to give 1000 mL for the day shift.
The nurse must document the actual amount of IV fluid given for the shift. Because the IV is behind, the patient will not receive 1000 mL for the shift.
e. Administer the IV fluid through an infusion pump.
The IV has been ordered to infuse via gravity. The nurse should assess the IV site to ensure proper placement.

Labeling IV Bags (pp. 92 – 94)

1.
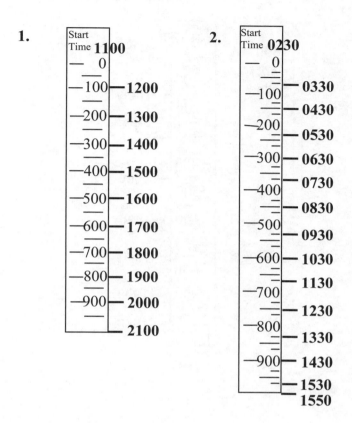

Start Time **1100**

— 0	
—100	—1200
—200	—1300
—300	—1400
—400	—1500
—500	—1600
—600	—1700
—700	—1800
—800	—1900
—900	—2000
	—2100

2.

Start Time **0230**

— 0	
—100	—0330
	—0430
—200	—0530
—300	—0630
—400	—0730
	—0830
—500	—0930
—600	—1030
	—1130
—700	—1230
—800	—1330
—900	—1430
	—1530
	1550

3.
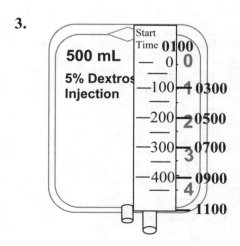

500 mL

5% Dextros Injection

Start Time **0100**

— 0	0
—100	0300
—200	0500
—300	0700
—400	0900
	1100

4.

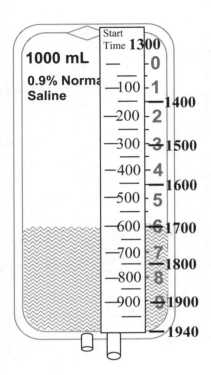

5.

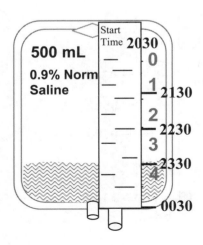

Exercise: FOCUS ON SAFETY
Making Clinical Judgments in Working With
Labeling IV Bags (p. 95)

> d. must be recalculated.
> **CORRECT:** *The nurse has made an error in the markings of the hourly fluid intake, beginning with the hourly fluid level at 1400. which should be at the 400 mL fluid level.*
>
> **INCORRECT:**
> b. is labeled appropriately.
> *There is an error with the hourly fluid level marking beginning at 1400.*
> c. reflects the increased rate.
> *The hourly fluid level intake is marked incorrectly on the flowmeter beginning at 1400.*
> c. indicates when the IV will be finished.
> *Since the hourly fluid level is not correct, the completion time is also incorrect.*

Module: PEDIATRIC CALCULATIONS

Working With Administering Medications to Children (pp. 96 – 99)

1.   2 tablets
2.   14 mL
3.   1.5 mL
4.   4 mL
5a. 2.5 mL
 b.

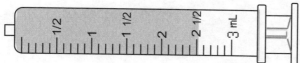

6a. 0.16 mL
 b.

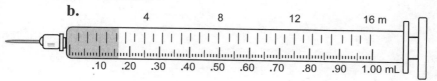

7. 1.2 mL
8a. 100 gtt / min
 b. 1430
9. 50 mL / hr

Dosage Based on Body Weight (pp. 100 – 102)
1a.   210 mg q.12h.
 b.   Yes, the dose is safe.
2a.   400 mcg / dose
 b.   Yes, the dose is safe.
3a.   180 mg / day
 b.   Yes, the dose is safe.
4a.   10.5 mg q.3–4h.
 b.   No, the dose is not safe.
5a.   73-147 mg / dose
 b.   Yes, the dose is safe.

Dosage Based on Body Surface Area (pp. 102 – 103)
1a.   5.6 mg q.6h.
 b.   Yes, the dose is safe.
2a.   198 mg / dose
 b.   No, the dose is not safe.
3a.   8.625 mg /q.1 – 2 weeks up to 12 weeks
 b.   No, the dose is not safe.
4a.   0.22 mg / day
 b.   Yes, the dose is safe.
5a.   590 mg q.8h. for 7 days
 b.   Yes, the dose is safe.

Exercise: FOCUS ON SAFETY
Making Clinical Judgments in Working With
Determining Safe Dose (p. 104)

b. question the ordered dose.

CORRECT: *The recommended total daily initial dose for a child weighing 27 kg is 35.64 mg / day. The order is for 40 mg b.i.d.*

INCORRECT:
a. administer the medication as ordered.
The nurse should first question the ordered dose, since it is more than the recommended initial dose.
c. ask the pharmacist if the ordered dose is correct.
The nurse should communicate directly with the physician and clarify the ordered dose.
e. ask the parent what dose the child has been taking.
The situation indicates that the physician is starting lamotrigine drug therapy on the child.

Working With Nastrogastric Fluid Replacement (pp. 105 – 107)

1a. 100 mL / hr
 b. 150 mL / hr
 c. 7 hours 36 minutes
 d. 2236 or 10:36 PM
2a. 63 mL / hr
 b. 22 mL / hr
 c. 3 hours
 d. 1500 or 3:00 PM
3a. 4 hours
 b. 0830 or 8:30 AM
4a. 4 hours 30 minutes
 b. 0315 or 3:15 AM
5a. 2 hours 36 minutes
 b. 1836 or 6:36 PM
6a. 3 hours 17 minutes
 b. 1017 or 10:17 AM

Module: TITRATION OF IV MEDICATIONS

Titration Problems in Common Clinical Practice (pp. 108 – 109)

1. 10 mL / hr
2. 20 mL / hr
3. 100 mg / hr
4. 35 mL / hr
5. 6 mL / hr
6a. 55 mL / hr
  b. 66 mL / hr

Complex Titration Problems in Critical Care (pp. 109 – 112)

1. a. 6 mg / hr
  b. 6 mL / hr
  c. No
2. a. 60 mg / hr
  b. 15 mL / hr
  c. 30 mL / hr
3. a. 120 mL / hr
  b. 60 mL / hr
4. 68 mL / hr
5. 60 mg / hr
6. 4 mg / min
7. 56 mL / hr
8. 3 mL / hr
9. 38 mL / hr
10. 30 mL / hr
11. 120 mL / hr
12. 12 mL / hr
13. 33 mL / hr
14. a. Yes
  b. 51 mL / hr

Exercise: FOCUS ON SAFETY
Making Clinical Judgments in Working With Titration (p. 113)

a. Set the infusion rate at 28 mL / hr.

CORRECT: *After calculating, the nurse will infuse the heparin at 28 mL / hr.*

d. Set-up the IV using an infusion pump.

CORRECT: *The nurse will infuse the heparin at 28 mL / hr using an infusion pump.*

INCORRECT:
b. set the infusion rate at _____ gtt / min.
Heparin is a high alert drug. It is safer to administer this drug through an infusion pump (mL / hr).
c. use a minidrop IV tubing for gravity flow infusion.
Heparin is a high alert drug. Therefore, every effort must be made to ensure accuracy in the administration of the ordered dose. An infusion pump accurately delivers the set rate.
e. discontinue the IV once the 500 mL have infused.
This is a continuous infusion and should not be discontinued without the physician's order.

Appendix

Body Surface Area Nomograms for Children

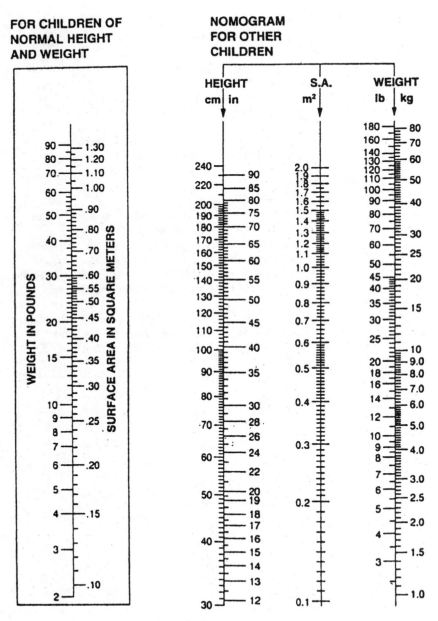

FOR CHILDREN OF NORMAL HEIGHT AND WEIGHT

NOMOGRAM FOR OTHER CHILDREN

(In Behrman RE, Vaughan VC, eds. *Nelson Textbook of Pediatrics*, 16th ed. Philadelphia, PA: WB Saunders Co., 2000.)